The

# Complete
# Mind Diet
## Cookbook for Over 50

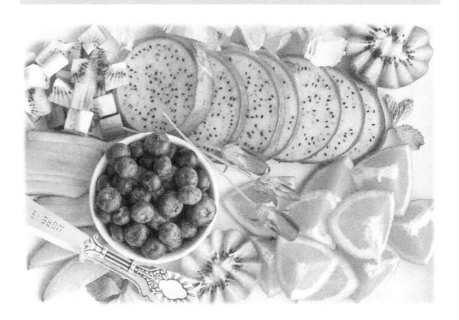

## Eric A. Randell

# COPYRIGHT

*SCAN HERE FOR MORE BOOKS FROM ME*

# TABLE OF CONTENTS

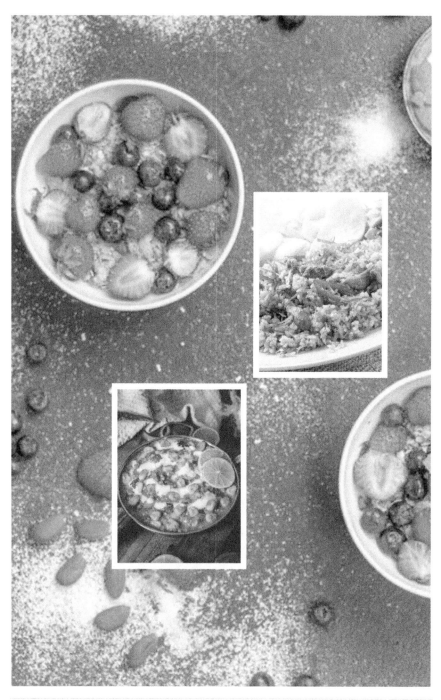

## INTRODUCTION

The importance of a balanced diet cannot be emphasized in an era when dementia diagnoses are on the rise. The Mind Diet Cookbook is a guide to keeping and safeguarding cognitive function, not just a compilation of tasty and healthy meals.

According to the World Health Organization, about 50 million individuals worldwide have dementia, with nearly 10 million new cases diagnosed each year. Because there is no known treatment, the emphasis has switched to prevention, and a nutritious diet is one of the most effective strategies to protect against dementia.

Numerous studies have shown that particular meals can have a major influence on brain function. The Mind Diet, which stands for "Mediterranean-DASH Intervention for Neurodegenerative Delay,"

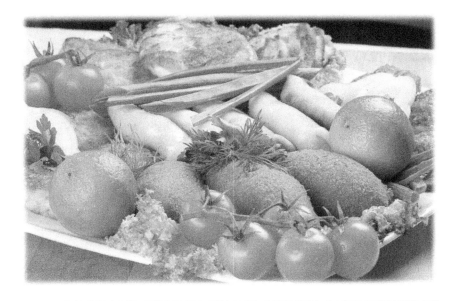

encourages the consumption of fruits, vegetables, whole grains, lean meats, and healthy fats. These meals are beneficial to both heart and brain health since they have been demonstrated to reduce the risk of cognitive decline and dementia.

According to studies, adopting the Mind Diet principles into your everyday life can potentially lower your chance of acquiring dementia by up to 35%. This is an eye-opening statistic that emphasizes the need to prioritize good nutrition.

The Mind Diet Cookbook is an excellent resource for anybody looking to improve their brain health. This cookbook presents a guide to greater brain health via the power of diet, with over 100 tasty and easy-to-follow recipes. This cookbook contains something for everyone, whether you want to eat more veggies or minimize your intake of processed foods.

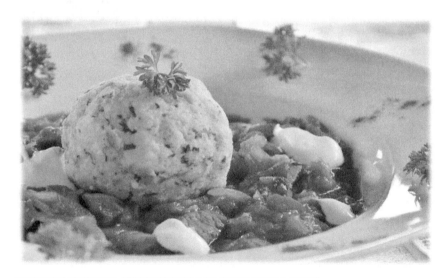

Incorporating a Mind Diet into your life is about living a longer, healthier, and more meaningful life, not merely preventing dementia. So, join us on this wonderful meal-by-meal journey to greater brain health.

## DEMENTIA EXPLAINED

Dementia is defined as the loss of cognitive functioning — thinking, remembering, and reasoning — to the point where it interferes with a person's everyday activities. Some persons with dementia lose control of their emotions, and their personalities may shift. Dementia fluctuates in intensity from moderate to severe, with the mildest stage affecting a person's functioning and the most severe level requiring the person to rely entirely on others for basic everyday functions.

Dementia affects millions of individuals and becomes more frequent as people age (approximately one-third of all persons aged 85 and older may have some kind of dementia), yet it is not a natural component of aging. A lot of people live to their 90s and over without any signs of dementia.

## HOW DOES FOOD HELP THE BRAIN?

Researchers are continuing to look at possible links between food and cognitive health. There is rising interest in Alzheimer's as a metabolic illness affecting the brain, as well as the involvement of Alzheimer's biomarkers, which are detectable indicators of biological processes in the body such as glucose metabolism. Researchers are looking at different diets, as well as particular foods and nutrients, in addition to the Mediterranean diet and its variants.

The ketogenic diet, for instance, is a high-fat, low-carbohydrate diet that stimulates the creation of ketones, molecules that assist brain cells' function. A study in animal and human tissue models found that a ketogenic diet may help brain cells use energy more efficiently, hence enhancing overall performance. A recent small pilot research of ten volunteers who followed a keto diet for three months found a statistically significant increase in cognition test results.

Several studies have found that treating and lowering high blood pressure can lessen the risk of dementia. Similar to the Mediterranean diet, the MIND diet emphasizes vegetables, particularly green leafy vegetables, berries over other fruits, healthy grains, legumes, nuts, one or more servings of fish per week, and olive oil. It also restricts the amount of red meat, sweets, cheese, butter/margarine, and fast/fried food that can be consumed.

Some, but not all, empirical research has found that the Mediterranean and MIND diets are linked to a decreased incidence of dementia when compared to a Western-style diet high in red meat, saturated fats, and sugar.

According to research, what you eat may affect your capacity which will optimize the memory function. Following an eating plan that includes a healthy selection of dietary fats and a range of plant foods high in phytonutrients may benefit your health. Phytonutrients are chemicals found in plants that are thought to be good for human health and can help avoid certain illnesses.

## WHAT TO EAT

There is still a lot to learn about what constitutes a brain-healthy diet. Studies show that what is beneficial for your heart may also be excellent for your brain. So, the greatest chance for rich memories is to avoid bad fats and vary your plant-based dietary intake.

### *Here are several diets that improve memory functioning.*

- Fruits
- Vegetables
- Whole grains and legumes
- Fish

- Healthier fats
- Herbs or seeds

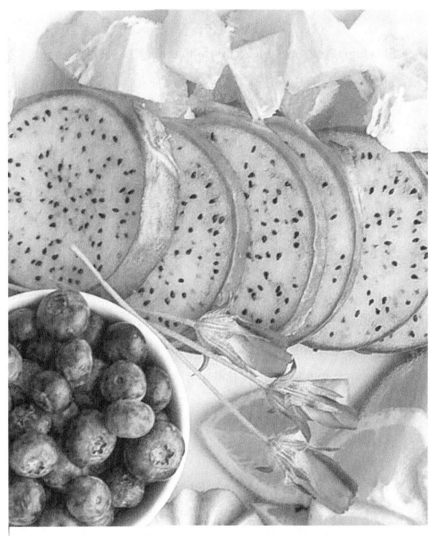

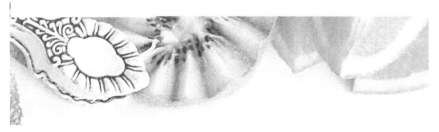

## BREAKFAST RECIPES

# Blueberry Chia Pudding

**Servings: 2 | Prep Time: 5 mins | Freezing Time: Overnight**

*Ingredients:*

- 1/2 cup chia seeds
- 2 cups almond milk
- 1 tablespoon honey
- 1/2 teaspoon vanilla extract
- 1/2 cup fresh blueberries

*Instructions:*

- ✓ In a bowl, mix chia seeds, almond milk, honey, and vanilla.
- ✓ Stir well and let it sit in the fridge overnight.
- ✓ Before serving, layer chia pudding with fresh blueberries.
- ✓ Enjoy a nutritious breakfast!

*Nutritional Information:*

*Calories: 220 | Protein: 7g | Fat: 10g | Carbs: 25g | Fiber: 12g*

# Veggie Breakfast Burritos

**Servings: 4 | Prep Time: 15 mins | Cooking Time: 10 mins**

*Ingredients:*

- 4 large eggs, beaten
- 1 cup black beans, nicely washed and drained
- 1 cup diced bell peppers
- 1 cup diced tomatoes
- 1 cup shredded cheddar cheese
- 4 whole wheat tortillas
- Salt and pepper to taste

*Instructions:*

- ✓ In a skillet, scramble the eggs until cooked.
- ✓ Add black beans, bell peppers, and tomatoes. Cook for 2-3 minutes.
- ✓ Warm tortillas and place egg mixture on each.
- ✓ Sprinkle cheese and fold into burritos.
- ✓ Serve warm for a hearty breakfast!

*Nutritional Information:*

*Calories: 320 | Protein: 18g | Fat: 14g | Carbs: 30g | Fiber: 8g*

## Greek Yogurt Parfait

**Servings: 2 | Prep Time: 5 mins | Cooking Time: 0 min**

*Ingredients:*

- 1 cup Greek yogurt
- 1/2 cup granola
- 1/2 cup mixed berries
- 2 tablespoons honey or maple syrup

*Instructions:*

- ✓ In serving glasses, layer Greek yogurt, granola, and berries.
- ✓ Nicely drizzle the honey or the maple syrup on top.
- ✓ Repeat layers.
- ✓ Serve chilled for a refreshing breakfast!

*Nutritional Information:*

*Calories: 280 | Protein: 15g | Fat: 8g | Carbs: 40g | Fiber: 6g*

## Spinach and Feta Omelet

**Servings: 2 | Prep Time: 10 mins | Cooking Time: 5 mins**

*Ingredients:*

- 4 large eggs

- 1 cup fresh spinach, chopped
- 1/4 cup crumbled feta cheese
- Salt and pepper to taste
- 1 tablespoon olive oil

*Instructions:*

- ✓ Beat eggs in a bowl and season with salt and pepper.
- ✓ Gently heat the olive oil in a skillet over moderate heat.
- ✓ Pour in beaten eggs and cook for 1 minute.
- ✓ Add spinach and feta on one half of the omelet.
- ✓ Fold the other half over the filling and cook for 2 minutes.
- ✓ Serve hot with a side of toast.

*Nutritional Information:*

*Calories: 250 | Protein: 18g | Fat: 18g | Carbs: 3g | Fiber: 1g*

# Banana Pancakes

**Servings: 2 | Prep Time: 10 mins | Cooking Time: 10 mins**

*Ingredients:*

- 2 ripe bananas, mashed
- 2 eggs
- 1/2 teaspoon vanilla extract

- 1/2 cup rolled oats
- 1/2 teaspoon cinnamon
- Butter or oil for cooking

*Instructions:*

- ✓ In a bowl, mix mashed bananas, eggs, and vanilla.
- ✓ Stir in rolled oats and cinnamon until combined.
- ✓ Heat butter or oil in a pan over medium heat.
- ✓ Pour small amounts of batter onto the pan.
- ✓ Cook for two (2) to three (3) minutes per side until golden.
- ✓ Serve warm with a drizzle of honey or fruit.

*Nutritional Information:*

*Calories: 270 | Protein: 10g | Fat: 9g | Carbs: 38g | Fiber: 5g*

# Apple Cinnamon Overnight Oats

**Servings: 2 | Prep Time: 5 mins | Freezing Time: Overnight**

*Ingredients:*

- 1 cup rolled oats
- 1 cup almond milk
- 1 apple, diced
- 1 tablespoon maple syrup

- 1/2 teaspoon cinnamon
- Chopped nuts for topping (optional)

*Instructions:*

✓ In a jar or bowl, combine oats, almond milk, diced apple, maple syrup, and cinnamon.

✓ Mix well, cover, and refrigerate overnight.

✓ In the morning, stir well and top with chopped nuts if desired.

✓ Enjoy a hassle-free, nutritious breakfast!

*Nutritional Information:*

*Calories: 290 | Protein: 7g | Fat: 5g | Carbs: 55g | Fiber: 8g*

# Breakfast Quinoa Bowl

**Servings: 2 | Prep Time: 10 mins | Cooking Time: 15 mins**

*Ingredients:*

- 1 cup quinoa, rinsed
- 2 cups water or vegetable broth
- 1 cup mixed berries
- 1/4 cup almonds, chopped
- 2 tablespoons honey or agave syrup

- Dash of cinnamon

*Instructions:*

✓ In a saucepan, bring quinoa and water/broth to a boil.

✓ Reduce heat, cover, and simmer for 12-15 minutes until quinoa is cooked.

✓ Divide cooked quinoa into bowls.

✓ Top with mixed berries, chopped almonds, a drizzle of honey/agave, and a dash of cinnamon.

✓ Enjoy a protein-packed breakfast bowl!

*Nutritional Information:*

*Calories: 320 | Protein: 10g | Fat: 8g | Carbs: 55g | Fiber: 7g*

## Peanut Butter Banana Toast

**Servings: 2 | Prep Time: 10 mins | Cooking Time: 5 mins**

*Ingredients:*

- 4 slices whole-grain bread
- 2 ripe bananas, sliced
- 4 tablespoons peanut butter
- Optional: honey or chia seeds for topping

*Instructions:*

✓ Toast the bread slices until golden.

✓ Spread peanut butter evenly on each slice.

✓ Top with banana slices.

✓ Optionally, drizzle honey or sprinkle chia seeds on top.

✓ Enjoy this simple yet satisfying breakfast!

*Nutritional Information:*

*Calories: 320 | Protein: 10g | Fat: 12g | Carbs: 45g | Fiber: 8g*

# Spinach and Tomato Breakfast Wrap

**Servings: 2 | Prep Time: 10 mins | Cooking Time: 5 mins**

*Ingredients:*

- 4 large eggs
- 1 cup fresh spinach leaves
- 1 tomato, sliced
- 1/2 cup shredded mozzarella cheese
- 2 whole wheat tortillas
- Salt and pepper to taste

*Instructions:*

- ✓ In a bowl, beat eggs and adjust with a little salt and pepper to your preferred taste.
- ✓ Heat a skillet over medium heat and scramble the eggs.
- ✓ Lay out tortillas and divide scrambled eggs onto each.
- ✓ Top with spinach, tomato slices, and shredded mozzarella.
- ✓ Roll up the tortillas into wraps.
- ✓ Warm in the skillet for 1-2 minutes on each side.
- ✓ Serve warm for a wholesome breakfast!

*Nutritional Information:*

*Calories: 320 | Protein: 18g | Fat: 15g | Carbs: 30g | Fiber: 6g*

# Breakfast Berry Smoothie

**Servings: 2 | Prep Time: 5 mins | Cooking Time: 0 min**

*Ingredients:*

- 1 cup mixed berries
- 1 ripe banana
- 1 cup Greek yogurt
- 1/2 cup almond milk
- 1 tablespoon honey or maple syrup (optional)

*Instructions:*

✓ Blend the mixed berries, banana, Greek yogurt, and almond milk until smooth.

✓ Add the honey or the maple syrup if additional sweetness is desired.

✓ Gently transfer into glasses and serve immediately.

*Nutritional Information:*

*Calories: 180 | Protein: 10g | Fat: 2g | Carbs: 35g | Fiber: 6g*

# Breakfast Egg Muffins

**Servings: 6 | Prep Time: 10 mins | Cooking Time: 20 mins**

*Ingredients:*

- 6 large eggs
- 1/2 cup diced bell peppers
- 1/2 cup chopped spinach
- 1/4 cup diced onions
- 1/2 cup shredded cheddar cheese
- Salt and pepper to taste

*Instructions:*

✓ Preheat the oven to 350°F (175°C) and grease a muffin tin.

✓ In a bowl, whisk eggs and adjust with a little salt and pepper to your preferred taste.

✓ Divide bell peppers, spinach, onions, and cheese among the muffin cups.

✓ Pour egg mixture into each cup until 3/4 full.

✓ Bake for 15-20 minutes until set.

✓ Let cool slightly before removing from the tin.

✓ Enjoy these convenient grab-and-go breakfast muffins!

*Nutritional Information:*

*Calories: 120 | Protein: 9g | Fat: 8g | Carbs: 3g | Fiber: 1g*

# Breakfast Stuffed Sweet Potatoes

**Servings: 2 | Prep Time: 10 mins | Cooking Time: 45 mins**

*Ingredients:*

- 2 medium sweet potatoes
- 4 strips bacon, cooked and crumbled
- 4 large eggs
- 1/2 cup diced tomatoes
- 1/4 cup chopped green onions
- Salt and pepper to taste

*Instructions:*

- ✓ Preheat the oven to 400°F (200°C).
- ✓ Pierce sweet potatoes with a fork and bake for 40-45 minutes until tender.
- ✓ While potatoes bake, scramble the eggs and season with salt and pepper.
- ✓ Once sweet potatoes are cooked, slice them open and fluff the insides.
- ✓ Fill each potato with scrambled eggs, diced tomatoes, bacon, and green onions.
- ✓ Serve hot for a hearty breakfast!

*Nutritional Information:*

*Calories: 380 | Protein: 20g | Fat: 18g | Carbs: 30g | Fiber: 5g*

## Coconut Chia Seed Pudding

**Servings: 2 | Prep Time: 5 mins | Freezing Time: Overnight**

*Ingredients:*

- 1/4 cup chia seeds
- 1 cup coconut milk
- 1 tablespoon honey or maple syrup
- 1/2 teaspoon vanilla extract

- Sliced fruits for topping (e.g., mango, pineapple)

*Instructions:*

✓ In a bowl, mix chia seeds, coconut milk, honey/maple syrup, and vanilla.

✓ Stir well and refrigerate overnight or for at least 4 hours.

✓ Before serving, stir the mixture to avoid clumps.

✓ Top with sliced fruits for a tropical twist!

*Nutritional Information:*

*Calories: 280 | Protein: 5g | Fat: 20g | Carbs: 20g | Fiber: 10g*

# Veggie Frittata

**Servings: 4 | Prep Time: 10 mins | Cooking Time: 25 mins**

*Ingredients:*

- 8 large eggs
- 1 cup diced bell peppers
- 1 cup diced zucchini
- 1 cup cherry tomatoes, halved
- 1/2 cup shredded mozzarella cheese
- Salt and pepper to taste

*Instructions:*

- ✓ Preheat the oven to 350°F (175°C).
- ✓ In a bowl, whisk eggs and adjust with a little salt and pepper to your preferred taste.
- ✓ Grease a baking dish and layer diced veggies.
- ✓ Pour whisked eggs over the veggies.
- ✓ Sprinkle shredded mozzarella on top.
- ✓ Bake for 20-25 minutes until eggs are set.
- ✓ Slice and serve this flavorful frittata!

*Nutritional Information:*

*Calories: 220 | Protein: 15g | Fat: 14g | Carbs: 8g | Fiber: 2g*

# Apple Cinnamon Breakfast Muffins

**Servings: 6 | Prep Time: 10 mins | Cooking Time: 20 mins**

*Ingredients:*

- 1 1/2 cups rolled oats
- 2 ripe bananas, mashed
- 1/2 cup unsweetened applesauce
- 1/4 cup almond milk

- 1 teaspoon cinnamon
- 1 teaspoon baking powder
- 1/2 teaspoon vanilla extract
- 1 apple, diced

*Instructions:*

✓ Preheat the oven to 375°F (190°C) and line a muffin tin with liners.
✓ In a bowl, mix rolled oats, mashed bananas, applesauce, almond milk, cinnamon, baking powder, and vanilla extract until combined.
✓ Gently fold in diced apple.
✓ Divide the batter into muffin cups.
✓ Bake for 18-20 minutes until golden and a toothpick comes out clean.
✓ Let cool before serving these wholesome apple-cinnamon muffins!

*Nutritional Information:*
*Calories: 150 | Protein: 3g | Fat: 2g | Carbs: 32g | Fiber: 4g*

# Breakfast Tacos

**Servings: 2 | Prep Time: 10 mins | Cooking Time: 5 mins**

*Ingredients:*

- 4 large eggs
- 4 small corn tortillas
- 1 avocado, sliced
- 1/2 cup black beans, drained and rinsed
- 1/2 cup salsa
- 1/4 cup chopped cilantro
- Salt and pepper to taste

*Instructions:*

- ✓ Scramble the eggs in a pan until cooked to your preference.
- ✓ Warm corn tortillas in a separate skillet or oven.
- ✓ Fill tortillas with scrambled eggs, avocado slices, black beans, salsa, and chopped cilantro.
- ✓ Season with salt and pepper.
- ✓ Serve these flavorful breakfast tacos!

*Nutritional Information:*

*Calories: 320 | Protein: 15g | Fat: 15g | Carbs: 35g | Fiber: 9g*

## Mediterranean Breakfast Bowl

**Servings: 2 | Prep Time: 10 mins | Cooking Time: 0 min**

*Ingredients:*

- 1 cup cooked quinoa
- 1/2 cup hummus
- 1 cucumber, diced
- 1 cup cherry tomatoes, halved
- 1/4 cup crumbled feta cheese
- 2 tablespoons chopped olives
- Fresh parsley for garnish

*Instructions:*

- ✓ Divide cooked quinoa into bowls.
- ✓ Top with dollops of hummus, diced cucumber, cherry tomatoes, feta cheese, and chopped olives.
- ✓ Garnish with fresh parsley.
- ✓ Enjoy this Mediterranean-inspired breakfast bowl!

*Nutritional Information:*

*Calories: 320 | Protein: 12g | Fat: 16g | Carbs: 35g | Fiber: 7g*

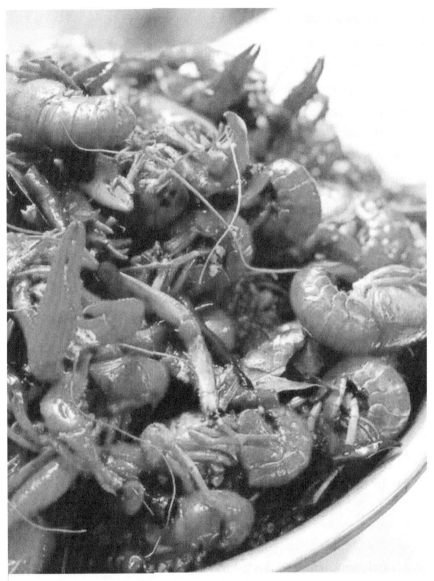

# FISH AND SEAFOOD RECIPES

## Garlic Butter Baked Cod

**Servings: 2 | Prep Time: 10 mins | Cooking Time: 15 mins**

*Ingredients:*

- 2 cod filets
- 2 tablespoons melted butter
- 2 cloves garlic, minced
- 1 tablespoon lemon juice
- 1 teaspoon paprika
- Salt and pepper to taste
- Fresh parsley for garnish

*Instructions:*

- ✓ Set the temperature of the oven to 400°F (200°C) and grease a baking dish.
- ✓ Pat dry the cod filets and place them in the baking dish.
- ✓ In a bowl, put together the melted butter, minced garlic, lemon juice, paprika, salt, and pepper.
- ✓ Pour the butter mixture over the cod filets.
- ✓ Bake for twelve (12) to fifteen (15) minutes until the fish flakes easily with a fork.
- ✓ Nicely garnish with fresh parsley before serving.

*Nutritional Information:*

*Calories: 250 | Protein: 30g | Fat: 12g | Carbs: 2g | Fiber: 0g*

# Grilled Shrimp Skewers

**Servings: 4 | Prep Time: 20 mins | Cooking Time: 6 mins**

*Ingredients:*

- 1-pound large shrimp, peeled with seeds removed
- 2 tablespoons olive oil
- 2 cloves garlic, minced
- 1 tablespoon lemon juice
- 1 teaspoon smoked paprika
- Salt and pepper to taste
- Wooden skewers, soaked in water

*Instructions:*

- ✓ In a bowl, put together the olive oil, minced garlic, lemon juice, paprika, salt, and pepper.
- ✓ Thread shrimp on skewers and brush with the marinade.
- ✓ Preheat the grill to moderate to high heat.
- ✓ Grill shrimp skewers for 2-3 minutes on each side until they turn pink and opaque.
- ✓ Serve hot, and enjoy these flavorful grilled shrimp skewers!

*Nutritional Information:*

*Calories: 160 | Protein: 25g | Fat: 7g | Carbs: 2g | Fiber: 0g*

## Lemon Herb Baked Salmon

**Servings: 2 | Prep Time: 10 mins | Cooking Time: 15 mins**

*Ingredients:*

- 2 salmon filets
- 2 tablespoons olive oil
- 2 tablespoons chopped fresh herbs
- Zest and juice of 1 lemon
- Salt and pepper to taste

*Instructions:*

- ✓ Set the temperature of the oven to 400°F (200°C) and line a baking sheet with parchment paper.
- ✓ Put the salmon filets on the prepared baking sheet.
- ✓ In a bowl, put together the olive oil, chopped herbs, lemon zest, lemon juice, salt, and pepper.
- ✓ Brush the herb mixture over the salmon filets.
- ✓ Bake for twelve (12) to fifteen (15) minutes until the salmon is cooked through.
- ✓ Serve immediately and savor this delightful lemon herb baked salmon!

*Nutritional Information:*

*Calories: 280 | Protein: 25g | Fat: 18g | Carbs: 1g | Fiber: 0g*

# Tuna Salad Stuffed Avocado

**Servings: 2 | Prep Time: 10 mins | Cooking Time: 0 min**

*Ingredients:*

- 2 cans (5 oz each) tuna
- 1/4 cup diced red onion
- 1/4 cup diced celery
- 2 tablespoons Greek yogurt
- 1 tablespoon lemon juice
- Salt and pepper to taste
- 2 avocados, halved and pitted
- Optional: chopped parsley for garnish

*Instructions:*

- ✓ In a bowl, put together the tuna, red onion, celery, Greek yogurt, lemon juice, salt, and pepper.
- ✓ Scoop out a bit of avocado flesh to create a larger cavity.
- ✓ Fill each avocado half with the tuna salad mixture.
- ✓ Garnish with chopped parsley if desired.
- ✓ Enjoy this protein-packed tuna salad served in avocado halves!

*Nutritional Information:*

*Calories: 280 | Protein: 25g | Fat: 15g | Carbs: 10g | Fiber: 7g*

# Cajun Shrimp Pasta

**Servings: 4 | Prep Time: 15 mins | Cooking Time: 15 mins**

*Ingredients:*

- 8 oz linguine pasta
- 1-pound large shrimp, peeled with veins removed
- 2 tablespoons olive oil
- 2 cloves garlic, minced
- 1 teaspoon Cajun seasoning
- 1 cup cherry tomatoes, halved
- 1/2 cup heavy cream
- Salt and pepper to taste
- Fresh parsley for garnish

*Instructions:*

- ✓ Cook linguine in accordance with the package instructions, then drain and set aside.
- ✓ In a skillet, heat olive oil over moderate heat.
- ✓ Add minced garlic and shrimp, sprinkle with Cajun seasoning. Cook for 2-3 minutes until shrimp turns pink.
- ✓ Add cherry tomatoes and cook for an additional 2 minutes.
- ✓ Pour in heavy cream, season with salt and pepper, and let it simmer for 2-3 minutes.
- ✓ Toss cooked linguine into the skillet and mix well.

✓ Garnish with fresh parsley before serving this delicious Cajun shrimp pasta!

*Nutritional Information:*

*Calories: 420 | Protein: 30g | Fat: 18g | Carbs: 35g | Fiber: 3g*

# Lemon Garlic Butter Scallops

**Servings: 2 | Prep Time: 10 mins | Cooking Time: 5 mins**

*Ingredients:*

- 10-12 large scallops
- 2 tablespoons butter
- 2 cloves garlic, minced
- Zest and juice of 1 lemon
- Salt and pepper to taste
- Chopped parsley for garnish

*Instructions:*

✓ Pat dry scallops and adjust with a little salt and pepper to your preferred taste.

✓ Heat butter in a skillet over moderate to high heat.

✓ Add minced garlic and cook for 30 seconds.

✓ Add scallops to the skillet and sear for 2-3 minutes per side until golden brown.

✓ Sprinkle lemon zest and drizzle lemon juice over the scallops.

✓ Nicely garnish with chopped parsley and serve immediately.

*Nutritional Information:*

*Calories: 200 | Protein: 25g | Fat: 8g | Carbs: 6g | Fiber: 0g*

# Baked Teriyaki Salmon

**Servings: 2 | Prep Time: 10 mins | Cooking Time: 15 mins**

*Ingredients:*

- 2 salmon filets
- 1/4 cup soy sauce
- 2 tablespoons honey
- 1 tablespoon rice vinegar
- 1 clove garlic, minced
- 1 teaspoon grated ginger
- Sesame seeds and chopped green onions for garnish

*Instructions:*

✓ Set the temperature of the oven to 400°F (200°C) and line a baking sheet with parchment paper.

✓ In a bowl, put together the soy sauce, honey, rice vinegar, minced garlic, and grated ginger.

✓ Put the salmon filets on the prepared baking sheet and brush with the teriyaki sauce.

✓ Bake for twelve (12) to fifteen (15) minutes until salmon is cooked through.

✓ Garnish with sesame seeds and chopped green onions before serving.

*Nutritional Information:*

*Calories: 280 | Protein: 25g | Fat: 12g | Carbs: 15g | Fiber: 0g*

# Baked Lemon Herb Tilapia

**Servings: 2 | Prep Time: 10 mins | Cooking Time: 15 mins**

*Ingredients:*

- 2 tilapia filets
- 2 tablespoons olive oil
- 2 cloves garlic, minced
- Zest and juice of 1 lemon
- 1 teaspoon dried mixed herbs
- Salt and pepper to taste
- Lemon slices for garnish

*Instructions:*

- ✓ Set the temperature of the oven to 400°F (200°C) and line a baking dish with parchment paper.
- ✓ Put the tilapia filets in the prepared dish.
- ✓ In a bowl, put together the olive oil, minced garlic, lemon zest, lemon juice, mixed herbs, salt, and pepper.
- ✓ Brush the herb mixture over the tilapia filets.
- ✓ Bake for twelve (12) to fifteen (15) minutes until the fish flakes easily with a fork.
- ✓ Garnish with lemon slices before serving.

*Nutritional Information:*

*Calories: 200 | Protein: 25g | Fat: 10g | Carbs: 2g | Fiber: 0.5g*

# Coconut Curry Shrimp

**Servings: 4 | Prep Time: 15 mins | Cooking Time: 15 mins**

*Ingredients:*

- 1-pound large shrimp, peeled with veins removed
- 1 tablespoon coconut oil
- 1 onion, diced
- 2 cloves garlic, minced

- 1 tablespoon curry powder
- 1 can (14 oz) coconut milk
- 1 red bell pepper, sliced
- Salt and pepper to taste
- Fresh cilantro for garnish

*Instructions:*

- ✓ Heat coconut oil in a pan over moderate heat.
- ✓ Add diced onion and minced garlic. Sauté for 2-3 minutes.
- ✓ Stir in curry powder and cook for another minute.
- ✓ Gently add the coconut milk and bring to a simmer.
- ✓ Add shrimp and sliced bell pepper, cook for 5-7 minutes until shrimp is cooked through.
- ✓ Season with salt and pepper.
- ✓ Garnish with fresh cilantro and serve this flavorful coconut curry shrimp!

*Nutritional Information:*

*Calories: 280 | Protein: 20g | Fat: 18g | Carbs: 10g | Fiber: 2g*

# Grilled Lemon Herb Swordfish

**Servings: 2 | Prep Time: 10 mins | Cooking Time: 10 mins**

*Ingredients:*

- 2 swordfish steaks
- 2 tablespoons olive oil
- Zest and juice of 1 lemon
- 1 teaspoon dried mixed herbs
- Salt and pepper to taste
- Lemon wedges for garnish

*Instructions:*

- ✓ Preheat the grill to moderate to high heat.
- ✓ In a bowl, put together the olive oil, lemon zest, lemon juice, mixed herbs, salt, and pepper.
- ✓ Brush the herb mixture onto both sides of the swordfish steaks.
- ✓ Grill swordfish for 4-5 minutes on each side until cooked through and grill marks appear.
- ✓ Serve with lemon wedges and enjoy this delightful grilled lemon herb swordfish!

*Nutritional Information:*

*Calories: 300 | Protein: 40g | Fat: 15g | Carbs: 1g | Fiber: 0.5g*

# Crispy Baked Coconut Shrimp

**Servings: 4 | Prep Time: 20 mins | Cooking Time: 15 mins**

*Ingredients:*

- 1-pound large shrimp, peeled with veins removed
- 1 cup shredded coconut
- 1/2 cup panko breadcrumbs
- 2 eggs, beaten
- Salt and pepper to taste
- Cooking spray

*Instructions:*

- ✓ Set the temperature of the oven to 400°F (200°C) and line a baking sheet with parchment paper.
- ✓ In one bowl, put together shredded coconut and panko breadcrumbs.
- ✓ Adjust the shrimp with a little salt and pepper to your preferred taste.
- ✓ Dip each shrimp in beaten eggs, then coat with the coconut breadcrumb mixture.
- ✓ Gently put coated shrimp on the prepared baking sheet.
- ✓ Lightly spray shrimp with cooking spray.
- ✓ Bake for twelve (12) to fifteen (15) minutes until the shrimp are golden and crispy.

✓ Serve with your favorite dipping sauce!

*Nutritional Information:*

*Calories: 280 | Protein: 25g | Fat: 15g | Carbs: 10g | Fiber: 2g*

# Grilled Teriyaki Tuna Steaks

**Servings: 2 | Prep Time: 15 mins | Cooking Time: 8 mins**

*Ingredients:*

- 2 tuna steaks
- 1/4 cup soy sauce
- 2 tablespoons honey
- 1 tablespoon rice vinegar
- 1 clove garlic, minced
- 1 teaspoon grated ginger
- Sesame seeds for garnish
- Sliced green onions for garnish

*Instructions:*

✓ In a bowl, whisk together the soy sauce, honey, rice vinegar, minced garlic, and grated ginger to create the teriyaki marinade.

✓ Marinate tuna steaks in the mixture for 10-15 minutes.

✓ Preheat the grill to moderate to high heat.

✓ Grill tuna steaks for 3-4 minutes per side until desired doneness.

✓ Sprinkle sesame seeds and sliced green onions on top.

✓ Serve these delicious grilled teriyaki tuna steaks!

*Nutritional Information:*

*Calories: 300 | Protein: 35g | Fat: 8g | Carbs: 20g | Fiber: 1g*

# Lemon Garlic Butter Lobster Tails

**Servings: 2 | Prep Time: 15 mins | Cooking Time: 10 mins**

*Ingredients:*

- 2 lobster tails
- 4 tablespoons butter
- 2 cloves garlic, minced
- Zest and juice of 1 lemon
- Salt and pepper to taste
- Chopped parsley for garnish

*Instructions:*

✓ Set the temperature of the oven to 425°F (220°C).

✓ Using kitchen shears, cut the top of the lobster shell lengthwise and pull the lobster meat upward.

✓ Melt butter in a small saucepan over low temperature.

✓ Add minced garlic, lemon zest, lemon juice, salt, and pepper to the melted butter.

✓ Brush the lobster tails generously with the garlic butter mixture.

✓ Bake for 8-10 minutes until lobster meat is opaque and cooked through.

✓ Garnish with chopped parsley and serve these flavorful lobster tails!

*Nutritional Information:*

*Calories: 250 | Protein: 30g | Fat: 15g | Carbs: 1g | Fiber: 0g*

# Baked Garlic Parmesan Crusted Halibut

**Servings: 2 | Prep Time: 15 mins | Cooking Time: 15 mins**

*Ingredients:*

- 2 halibut filets
- 1/4 cup grated Parmesan cheese
- 2 tablespoons melted butter
- 2 cloves garlic, minced
- 1/4 cup breadcrumbs
- 1 tablespoon chopped fresh parsley
- Salt and pepper to taste

- Lemon wedges for garnish

*Instructions:*

✓ Set the temperature of the oven to 400°F (200°C) and line a baking sheet with parchment paper.

✓ In a bowl, put together the grated Parmesan cheese, melted butter, minced garlic, breadcrumbs, chopped parsley, salt, and pepper.

✓ Gently put the halibut filets on the prepared baking sheet.

✓ Spread the Parmesan mixture evenly over the top of each filet, pressing gently to adhere.

✓ Bake for twelve (12) to fifteen (15) minutes until the fish is cooked through and the topping is golden brown.

✓ Serve with lemon wedges for a zesty touch!

*Nutritional Information:*

*Calories: 300 | Protein: 35g | Fat: 15g | Carbs: 5g | Fiber: 1g*

# Mediterranean Baked Sea Bass

**Servings: 2 | Prep Time: 15 mins | Cooking Time: 20 mins**

*Ingredients:*

- 2 sea bass filets

- 2 tablespoons olive oil
- 2 cloves garlic, minced
- 1 teaspoon dried oregano
- 1 teaspoon dried basil
- 1/2 cup cherry tomatoes, halved
- 1/4 cup Kalamata olives, pitted and divided in equal halves
- 2 tablespoons crumbled feta cheese
- Salt and pepper to taste
- Lemon wedges for garnish

*Instructions:*

✓ Set the temperature of the oven to 375°F (190°C) and line a baking dish with parchment paper.

✓ Gently place the sea bass filets in the prepared baking dish.

✓ In a bowl, put together the olive oil, minced garlic, oregano, basil, salt, and pepper.

✓ Spread the olive oil mixture over the sea bass filets.

✓ Top with cherry tomatoes, Kalamata olives, and crumbled feta cheese.

✓ Bake for 18-20 minutes until the fish is cooked and flakes easily.

✓ Garnish with lemon wedges before serving this Mediterranean delight!

*Nutritional Information:*

*Calories: 280 | Protein: 30g | Fat: 15g | Carbs: 5g | Fiber: 2g*

# Cajun Blackened Catfish

**Servings: 2 | Prep Time: 10 mins | Cooking Time: 10 mins**

*Ingredients:*

- 2 catfish filets
- 2 tablespoons Cajun seasoning
- 2 tablespoons olive oil
- 1 tablespoon butter
- Lemon wedges for garnish

*Instructions:*

- ✓ Rub Cajun seasoning evenly over both sides of the catfish filets.
- ✓ Heat olive oil and butter in a skillet over moderate to high heat.
- ✓ Once the skillet is hot, add the catfish filets.
- ✓ Cook for 4-5 minutes on each side until the fish is blackened and cooked through.
- ✓ Squeeze lemon juice over the catfish before serving.

*Nutritional Information:*

*Calories: 250 | Protein: 25g | Fat: 15g | Carbs: 2g | Fiber: 1g*

# Seared Scallops with Herb Butter

**Servings: 2 | Prep Time: 10 mins | Cooking Time: 5 mins**

*Ingredients:*

- 10-12 large scallops
- 2 tablespoons butter
- 2 cloves garlic, minced
- 1 tablespoon chopped fresh herbs
- Salt and pepper to taste
- Lemon wedges for garnish

*Instructions:*

- ✓ Pat dry scallops and adjust with a little salt and pepper to your preferred taste.
- ✓ Heat butter in a skillet over moderate to high heat.
- ✓ Add minced garlic and cook for 30 seconds.
- ✓ Add scallops to the skillet and sear for 2-3 minutes per side until golden brown.
- ✓ Sprinkle chopped fresh herbs over the scallops.
- ✓ Serve with lemon wedges for added freshness.

*Nutritional Information:*

*Calories: 200 | Protein: 25g | Fat: 10g | Carbs: 3g | Fiber: 0.5g*

# Shrimp and Veggie Stir-Fry

**Servings: 4 | Prep Time: 15 mins | Cooking Time: 10 mins**

*Ingredients:*

- 1-pound large shrimp, peeled with veins removed
- 2 tablespoons soy sauce
- 1 tablespoon hoisin sauce
- 1 tablespoon sesame oil
- 2 cloves garlic, minced
- 1 teaspoon grated ginger
- 1 bell pepper, sliced
- 1 cup broccoli florets
- 1 cup snow peas
- 2 green onions, sliced
- Cooked rice for serving

*Instructions:*

- ✓ In a bowl, put together the shrimp with soy sauce and hoisin sauce. Set aside to marinate.
- ✓ Heat sesame oil in a large skillet or wok over moderate to high heat.
- ✓ Add minced garlic and grated ginger, sauté for 30 seconds.
- ✓ Add marinated shrimp and cook for 2-3 minutes until pink.

✓ Add sliced bell pepper, broccoli florets, and snow peas. Stir-fry for 3-4 minutes until the veggies are tender-crisp.

✓ Sprinkle sliced green onions over the stir-fry.

✓ Serve over cooked rice and enjoy this vibrant shrimp and veggie stir-fry!

*Nutritional Information:*

*Calories: 220 | Protein: 25g | Fat: 5g | Carbs: 20g | Fiber: 4g*

## Grilled Lemon Garlic Swordfish

**Servings: 2 | Prep Time: 10 mins | Cooking Time: 10 mins**

*Ingredients:*

- 2 swordfish steaks
- 2 tablespoons olive oil
- Zest and juice of 1 lemon
- 2 cloves garlic, minced
- 1 teaspoon dried oregano
- Salt and pepper to taste
- Lemon wedges for garnish

*Instructions:*

✓ Preheat the grill to moderate to high heat.

✓ In a bowl, put together the olive oil, lemon zest, lemon juice, minced garlic, dried oregano, salt, and pepper.

✓ Brush the mixture over both sides of the swordfish steaks.

✓ Grill swordfish for 4-5 minutes on each side until cooked through and grill marks appear.

✓ Serve with lemon wedges and relish this delightful grilled lemon garlic swordfish!

*Nutritional Information:*

*Calories: 280 | Protein: 30g | Fat: 15g | Carbs: 2g | Fiber: 0.5g*

# Baked Herb Crusted Salmon

**Servings: 2 | Prep Time: 10 mins | Cooking Time: 15 mins**

*Ingredients:*

- 2 salmon filets
- 2 tablespoons Dijon mustard
- 1/4 cup breadcrumbs
- 1 tablespoon chopped fresh herbs
- 1 tablespoon olive oil
- Salt and pepper to taste
- Lemon wedges for garnish

*Instructions:*

✓ Set the temperature of the oven to 400°F (200°C) and line a baking sheet with parchment paper.

✓ Gently put the salmon filets on the prepared baking sheet.

✓ Spread Dijon mustard over the top of each filet.

✓ In a bowl, mix breadcrumbs, chopped fresh herbs, olive oil, salt, and pepper.

✓ Pat the breadcrumb mixture onto the mustard-coated salmon filets.

✓ Bake for twelve (12) to fifteen (15) minutes until the salmon is cooked through and the topping is golden brown.

✓ Serve with lemon wedges and enjoy this flavorful herb-crusted salmon!

*Nutritional Information:*

*Calories: 300 | Protein: 30g | Fat: 15g | Carbs: 10g | Fiber: 1g*

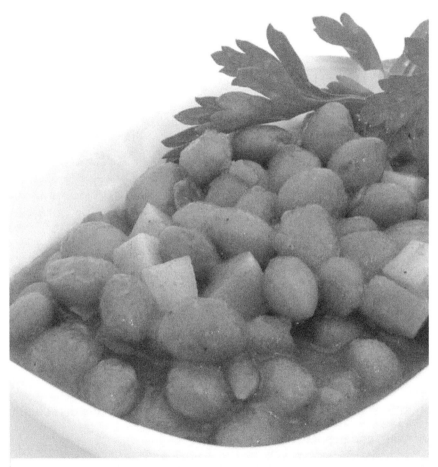

# BEANS, GRAINS, AND PASTA RECIPES

# Quinoa Stuffed Bell Peppers

**Servings: 4 | Prep Time: 15 mins | Cooking Time: 30 mins**

*Ingredients:*

- 4 bell peppers, tops removed and seeds carefully removed
- 1 cup quinoa, cooked
- 1 can (15 oz) black beans, carefully washed and drained
- 1 cup corn kernels
- 1 cup diced tomatoes
- 1/2 cup shredded cheddar cheese
- 1 teaspoon chili powder
- 1/2 teaspoon cumin
- Salt and pepper to taste
- Chopped cilantro for garnish

*Instructions:*

- ✓ Set the temperature of the oven to 375°F (190°C).
- ✓ In a bowl, put together the cooked quinoa, black beans, corn, diced tomatoes, shredded cheddar cheese, chili powder, cumin, salt, and pepper.
- ✓ Stuff each bell pepper with the quinoa mixture.
- ✓ Gently place the stuffed peppers in a baking dish.
- ✓ Cover with foil and bake for twenty-five (25) minutes.

✓ Remove foil and bake for an additional 5 minutes until peppers are tender and filling is heated through.

✓ Garnish with chopped cilantro before serving these delicious quinoa stuffed bell peppers!

*Nutritional Information:*

*Calories: 300 | Protein: 12g | Fat: 8g | Carbs: 45g | Fiber: 10g*

# Lentil and Vegetable Soup

**Servings: 6 | Prep Time: 15 mins | Cooking Time: 40 mins**

*Ingredients:*

- 1 cup dried lentils, rinsed
- 6 cups vegetable broth
- 1 onion, diced
- 2 carrots, diced
- 2 celery stalks, diced
- 2 cloves garlic, minced
- 1 can (14 oz) diced tomatoes
- 1 teaspoon dried thyme
- 1 teaspoon paprika
- Salt and pepper to taste
- Fresh parsley for garnish

*Instructions:*

✓ In a large pot, put together the lentils, vegetable broth, diced onion, carrots, celery, minced garlic, diced tomatoes, thyme, paprika, salt, and pepper.

✓ Bring to a boil, then reduce heat and simmer for 30-35 minutes until lentils and vegetables are tender.

✓ Adjust seasoning if needed.

✓ Ladle the lentil and vegetable soup into bowls.

✓ Garnish with fresh parsley before serving this comforting soup!

*Nutritional Information:*

*Calories: 220 | Protein: 14g | Fat: 1g | Carbs: 40g | Fiber: 12g*

# Spinach and Mushroom Risotto

**Servings: 4 | Prep Time: 10 mins | Cooking Time: 30 mins**

*Ingredients:*

- 1 1/2 cups Arborio rice
- 4 cups vegetable broth
- 1 onion, finely chopped
- 2 cloves garlic, minced
- 2 cups sliced mushrooms

- 3 cups fresh spinach leaves
- 1/2 cup grated Parmesan cheese
- 2 tablespoons olive oil
- Salt and pepper to taste
- Chopped parsley for garnish

*Instructions:*

✓ In a pot, gently heat the vegetable broth and keep it warm.

✓ In a separate large skillet, heat olive oil over moderate heat.

✓ Sauté chopped onion and minced garlic until translucent.

✓ Add Arborio rice to the skillet and cook for 1-2 minutes until the rice is slightly toasted.

✓ Gradually add warm vegetable broth, one ladle at a time, stirring constantly until absorbed.

✓ Stir in sliced mushrooms and continue adding broth until rice is creamy and cooked but slightly al dente.

✓ Fold in fresh spinach and grated Parmesan cheese until spinach wilts and cheese melts.

✓ Adjust with a little salt and pepper to your preferred taste.

✓ Garnish with chopped parsley before serving this creamy spinach and mushroom risotto!

*Nutritional Information:*

*Calories: 350 | Protein: 10g | Fat: 8g | Carbs: 60g | Fiber: 4g*

# Chickpea and Vegetable Stir-Fry

**Servings: 4 | Prep Time: 15 mins | Cooking Time: 15 mins**

*Ingredients:*

- 2 cups cooked chickpeas
- 1 red bell pepper, sliced
- 1 yellow bell pepper, sliced
- 1 cup broccoli florets
- 1 cup sliced carrots
- 1/4 cup soy sauce
- 2 tablespoons sesame oil
- 2 cloves garlic, minced
- 1 tablespoon grated ginger
- 2 green onions, sliced
- Cooked rice or quinoa for serving

*Instructions:*

- ✓ Heat sesame oil in a large skillet or wok over moderate to high heat.
- ✓ Add minced garlic and grated ginger, sauté for 30 seconds.
- ✓ Stir in sliced bell peppers, broccoli florets, and sliced carrots. Cook for three (3) to four (4) minutes until vegetables are tender-crisp.

✓ Add cooked chickpeas to the skillet and stir-fry for another 2-3 minutes.

✓ Pour soy sauce over the stir-fry and toss to coat evenly.

✓ Garnish with sliced green onions.

✓ Serve over cooked rice or quinoa for a delightful chickpea and vegetable stir-fry!

*Nutritional Information:*

*Calories: 280 | Protein: 10g | Fat: 8g | Carbs: 40g | Fiber: 10g*

# Pesto Pasta with Cherry Tomatoes
**Servings: 4 | Prep Time: 10 mins | Cooking Time: 15 mins**

*Ingredients:*

- 8 oz pasta (any pasta of choice such as spaghetti or penne)
- 1/2 cup basil pesto
- 1 cup cherry tomatoes, halved
- 1/4 cup grated Parmesan cheese
- 2 tablespoons pine nuts (optional)
- Salt and pepper to taste
- Fresh basil leaves for garnish

*Instructions:*

✓ Cook pasta in accordance with the package instructions, then drain and set aside.

✓ In a large bowl, toss the cooked pasta with basil pesto until well coated.

✓ Add cherry tomatoes and grated Parmesan cheese, mix gently.

✓ Toast pine nuts in a dry skillet over medium heat for a few minutes until golden (if using).

✓ Sprinkle toasted pine nuts over the pesto pasta.

✓ Adjust with a little salt and pepper to your preferred taste.

✓ Garnish with fresh basil leaves and serve this flavorful pesto pasta!

*Nutritional Information:*

*Calories: 350 | Protein: 10g | Fat: 15g | Carbs: 45g | Fiber: 3g*

# Black Bean and Corn Salad

**Servings: 6 | Prep Time: 10 mins | Cooking Time: 0 min**

*Ingredients:*

● 2 cans (15 oz each) black beans, carefully washed and drained

● 1 cup corn kernels (fresh, canned, or thawed frozen)

● 1 red bell pepper, diced

- 1/2 red onion, finely chopped
- 1/4 cup chopped fresh cilantro
- 2 tablespoons olive oil
- 2 tablespoons lime juice
- 1 teaspoon ground cumin
- Salt and pepper to taste
- Avocado slices for garnish (optional)

*Instructions:*

✓ In a large bowl, put together the black beans, corn kernels, diced red bell pepper, finely chopped red onion, and chopped fresh cilantro.

✓ In a separate small bowl, whisk together olive oil, lime juice, ground cumin, salt, and pepper.

✓ Transfer the dressing over the black bean mixture and toss gently to coat.

✓ Garnish with avocado slices if desired.

✓ Serve this vibrant black bean and corn salad as a refreshing side dish or light meal!

*Nutritional Information:*

*Calories: 200 | Protein: 8g | Fat: 6g | Carbs: 30g | Fiber: 8g*

# Mushroom Risotto

**Servings: 4 | Prep Time: 10 mins | Cooking Time: 30 mins**

*Ingredients:*

- 1 1/2 cups Arborio rice
- 4 cups vegetable broth
- 1 onion, finely chopped
- 2 cloves garlic, minced
- 2 cups sliced mushrooms
- 1/2 cup dry white wine
- 1/2 cup grated Parmesan cheese
- 2 tablespoons butter
- Salt and pepper to taste
- Chopped parsley for garnish

*Instructions:*

- ✓ In a pot, gently heat the vegetable broth and keep it warm.
- ✓ In a large skillet, melt butter over moderate heat.
- ✓ Sauté chopped onion and minced garlic until translucent.
- ✓ Add Arborio rice to the skillet and cook for 1-2 minutes until the rice is slightly toasted.
- ✓ Pour in dry white wine and stir until absorbed.
- ✓ Gradually add warm vegetable broth, one ladle at a time, stirring constantly until absorbed and rice is creamy but slightly al dente.

✓ Stir in sliced mushrooms and cook until mushrooms are tender.

✓ Fold in grated Parmesan cheese until melted and well combined.

✓ Adjust with a little salt and pepper to your preferred taste.

✓ Garnish with chopped parsley before serving this creamy mushroom risotto!

*Nutritional Information:*

*Calories: 350 | Protein: 8g | Fat: 10g | Carbs: 50g | Fiber: 3g*

# Lemon Garlic Pasta with Spinach

**Servings: 4 | Prep Time: 10 mins | Cooking Time: 15 mins**

*Ingredients:*

- 8 oz pasta (linguine or spaghetti)
- 3 cups fresh spinach leaves
- 3 tablespoons olive oil
- 4 cloves garlic, minced
- Zest and juice of 1 lemon
- 1/4 cup grated Parmesan cheese
- Salt and pepper to taste
- Red pepper flakes for garnish (optional)

*Instructions:*

- ✓ Cook pasta in accordance with the package instructions, then drain and set aside.
- ✓ Heat olive oil in a large skillet over moderate heat.
- ✓ Add minced garlic and sauté for 1-2 minutes until fragrant.
- ✓ Stir in fresh spinach leaves and cook until wilted.
- ✓ Add cooked pasta to the skillet.
- ✓ Add lemon zest and lemon juice, toss well to coat.
- ✓ Stir in grated Parmesan cheese until pasta is coated and creamy.
- ✓ Adjust with a little salt and pepper to your preferred taste.
- ✓ Garnish with red pepper flakes for a touch of heat if desired.
- ✓ Serve this zesty lemon garlic pasta with spinach for a delightful meal!

*Nutritional Information:*

*Calories: 300 | Protein: 8g | Fat: 10g | Carbs: 45g | Fiber: 3g*

# Butternut Squash Risotto

**Servings: 4 | Prep Time: 15 mins | Cooking Time: 30 mins**

*Ingredients:*

- 1 1/2 cups Arborio rice
- 4 cups vegetable broth

- 2 cups diced butternut squash
- 1 onion, finely chopped
- 2 cloves garlic, minced
- 1/2 cup dry white wine
- 1/4 cup grated Parmesan cheese
- 2 tablespoons butter
- 1 tablespoon olive oil
- Salt and pepper to taste
- Chopped sage leaves for garnish

*Instructions:*

✓ In a pot, gently heat the vegetable broth and keep it warm.

✓ In a separate large skillet, heat olive oil and butter over moderate heat.

✓ Sauté chopped onion and minced garlic until translucent.

✓ Add Arborio rice to the skillet and cook for 1-2 minutes until the rice is slightly toasted.

✓ Pour in dry white wine and stir until absorbed.

✓ Gradually add warm vegetable broth, one ladle at a time, stirring constantly until absorbed and rice is creamy but slightly al dente.

✓ Stir in diced butternut squash and continue adding broth until squash is tender and rice is creamy.

✓ Fold in grated Parmesan cheese until melted and well combined.

✓ Adjust with a little salt and pepper to your preferred taste.

✓ Garnish with chopped sage leaves before serving this comforting butternut squash risotto!

*Nutritional Information:*

*Calories: 320 | Protein: 7g | Fat: 10g | Carbs: 50g | Fiber: 3g*

## Pasta Primavera

**Servings: 4 | Prep Time: 15 mins | Cooking Time: 15 mins**

*Ingredients:*

- 8 oz pasta (any pasta of choice such as penne or fettuccine)
- 2 cups assorted vegetables
- 2 cloves garlic, minced
- 1/4 cup olive oil
- 1/4 cup grated Parmesan cheese
- 1 tablespoon chopped fresh basil
- 1 tablespoon chopped fresh parsley
- Salt and pepper to taste

*Instructions:*

✓ Cook pasta in accordance with the package instructions, then drain and set aside.

✓ In a large skillet, heat olive oil over moderate heat.

✓ Add minced garlic and sauté for 1-2 minutes until fragrant.

✓ Add assorted vegetables to the skillet and cook for 5-7 minutes until tender-crisp.

✓ Toss cooked pasta into the skillet with the vegetables.

✓ Stir in grated Parmesan cheese, chopped fresh basil, and chopped fresh parsley.

✓ Adjust with a little salt and pepper to your preferred taste.

✓ Serve this vibrant pasta primavera for a delightful and colorful dish!

*Nutritional Information:*

*Calories: 320 | Protein: 8g | Fat: 12g | Carbs: 45g | Fiber: 4g*

# Spaghetti Aglio e Olio

**Servings: 4 | Prep Time: 10 mins | Cooking Time: 15 mins**

*Ingredients:*

- 8 oz spaghetti
- 1/4 cup olive oil
- 6 cloves garlic, thinly sliced
- 1/2 teaspoon red pepper flakes
- 1/4 cup chopped fresh parsley
- Grated Parmesan cheese for garnish

- Salt to taste

*Instructions:*

✓ Cook spaghetti in accordance with the package instructions, then drain and set aside.

✓ In a large skillet, heat olive oil over moderate low heat.

✓ Add thinly sliced garlic and red pepper flakes to the skillet.

✓ Cook for 3-4 minutes until garlic turns golden but not browned.

✓ Add cooked spaghetti to the skillet and toss to coat with the garlic-infused oil.

✓ Stir in chopped fresh parsley and season with salt.

✓ Serve this simple yet flavorful spaghetti aglio e olio with grated Parmesan cheese on top!

*Nutritional Information:*

*Calories: 300 | Protein: 8g | Fat: 14g | Carbs: 35g | Fiber: 2g*

# Lentil Shepherd's Pie

**Servings: 6 | Prep Time: 20 mins | Cooking Time: 40 mins**

*Ingredients:*

- 2 cups cooked lentils
- 1 onion, diced

- 2 carrots, diced
- 1 cup peas (fresh or frozen)
- 2 cloves garlic, minced
- 1 cup vegetable broth
- 2 tablespoons tomato paste
- 1 teaspoon Worcestershire sauce (optional)
- 4 cups mashed potatoes
- Salt and pepper to taste
- Chopped fresh parsley for garnish

*Instructions:*

✓ Set the temperature of the oven to 375°F (190°C).

✓ In a skillet, sauté diced onion and diced carrots until softened.

✓ Add minced garlic and cook for 1 minute.

✓ Stir in cooked lentils, peas, vegetable broth, tomato paste, and Worcestershire sauce (if using). Cook for 5-7 minutes until heated through and slightly thickened.

✓ Gently transfer the lentil mixture to a baking dish.

✓ Spread mashed potatoes over the lentil mixture.

✓ Bake for twenty-five (25) to thirty (30) minutes until the top is golden brown.

✓ Garnish with chopped fresh parsley before serving this hearty lentil shepherd's pie!

*Nutritional Information:*

*Calories: 280 | Protein: 10g | Fat: 5g | Carbs: 50g | Fiber: 10g*

# Veggie-Packed Spaghetti Bolognese

**Servings: 4 | Prep Time: 15 mins | Cooking Time: 30 mins**

*Ingredients:*

- 8 oz spaghetti
- 1 onion, finely chopped
- 2 carrots, diced
- 2 celery stalks, diced
- 2 cloves garlic, minced
- 1 cup mushrooms, sliced
- 1 can (14 oz) crushed tomatoes
- 1 tablespoon tomato paste
- 1 teaspoon dried oregano
- 1 teaspoon dried basil
- Salt and pepper to taste
- Grated Parmesan cheese for garnish
- Chopped fresh basil for garnish

*Instructions:*

✓ Cook spaghetti in accordance with the package instructions, then drain and set aside.

✓ In a large skillet, sauté chopped onion, diced carrots, and diced celery until softened.

✓ Add minced garlic and sliced mushrooms, cook for 2-3 minutes.

✓ Stir in crushed tomatoes, tomato paste, dried oregano, dried basil, salt, and pepper.

✓ Simmer for 15-20 minutes until the sauce thickens.

✓ Serve the veggie-packed Bolognese sauce over cooked spaghetti.

✓ Garnish with grated Parmesan cheese and chopped fresh basil.

*Nutritional Information:*

*Calories: 320 | Protein: 10g | Fat: 3g | Carbs: 60g | Fiber: 8g*

# Red Lentil Curry

**Servings: 4 | Prep Time: 10 mins | Cooking Time: 25 mins**

*Ingredients:*

● 1 cup red lentils, rinsed

● 1 onion, finely chopped

● 2 cloves garlic, minced

- 1 tablespoon grated ginger
- 1 can (14 oz) coconut milk
- 1 can (14 oz) diced tomatoes
- 2 tablespoons curry powder
- 1 teaspoon turmeric
- 1 teaspoon cumin
- 1 teaspoon paprika
- Salt and pepper to taste
- Fresh cilantro for garnish
- Cooked rice for serving

*Instructions:*

- ✓ In a pot, put together the red lentils, chopped onion, minced garlic, grated ginger, coconut milk, diced tomatoes, curry powder, turmeric, cumin, paprika, salt, and pepper.
- ✓ Bring to a boil, then reduce heat and simmer for 20-25 minutes until lentils are tender and the curry thickens.
- ✓ Adjust seasoning if needed.
- ✓ Serve the flavorful red lentil curry over cooked rice.
- ✓ Garnish with fresh cilantro before serving.

*Nutritional Information:*

*Calories: 280 | Protein: 15g | Fat: 10g | Carbs: 35g | Fiber: 12g*

# Three Bean Chili

**Servings: 6 | Prep Time: 15 mins | Cooking Time: 30 mins**

*Ingredients:*

- 1 can (15 oz) black beans, carefully washed and drained
- 1 can (15 oz) kidney beans, carefully washed and drained
- 1 can (15 oz) cannellini beans, carefully washed and drained
- 1 onion, chopped
- 2 cloves garlic, minced
- 1 bell pepper, diced
- 1 can (14 oz) diced tomatoes
- 2 cups vegetable broth
- 2 tablespoons chili powder
- 1 teaspoon cumin
- 1 teaspoon paprika
- Salt and pepper to taste
- Chopped fresh cilantro for garnish
- Sour cream (optional) for topping

*Instructions:*

- ✓ In a large pot, sauté chopped onion, minced garlic, and diced bell pepper until softened.

✓ Add black beans, kidney beans, cannellini beans, diced tomatoes, vegetable broth, chili powder, cumin, paprika, salt, and pepper to the pot.

✓ Bring to a boil, then reduce heat and simmer for twenty (20) to twenty-five (25) minutes.

✓ Adjust seasoning if needed.

✓ Serve the hearty three bean chili topped with chopped fresh cilantro and a dollop of sour cream if desired.

*Nutritional Information:*

*Calories: 250 | Protein: 15g | Fat: 1g | Carbs: 45g | Fiber: 15g*

# Mushroom and Spinach Stuffed Shells

**Servings: 4 | Prep Time: 20 mins | Cooking Time: 25 mins**

*Ingredients:*

- 16 jumbo pasta shells, cooked according to package instructions
- 2 cups ricotta cheese
- 1 cup chopped spinach
- 1 cup chopped mushrooms
- 1/2 cup grated Parmesan cheese
- 1 egg, beaten

- 1 teaspoon dried basil
- 1 teaspoon dried oregano
- Salt and pepper to taste
- 2 cups marinara sauce
- Shredded mozzarella cheese for topping

*Instructions:*

✓ Set the temperature of the oven to 375°F (190°C).
✓ In a bowl, mix the ricotta cheese, chopped spinach, chopped mushrooms, grated Parmesan cheese, beaten egg, dried basil, dried oregano, salt, and pepper.
✓ Stuff each cooked pasta shell with the ricotta mixture.
✓ Spread marinara sauce in a baking dish.
✓ Place stuffed shells in the dish over the sauce.
✓ Top with shredded mozzarella cheese.
✓ Bake for 20-25 minutes until the cheese is bubbly and golden.
✓ Serve these delightful mushroom and spinach stuffed shells!

*Nutritional Information:*
*Calories: 380 | Protein: 20g | Fat: 15g | Carbs: 40g | Fiber: 4g*

# Chickpea and Quinoa Salad

**Servings: 4 | Prep Time: 15 mins | Cooking Time: 15 mins**

*Ingredients:*

- 1 cup quinoa, cooked
- 1 can (15 oz) chickpeas, carefully washed and drained
- 1 cucumber, diced
- 1 red bell pepper, diced
- 1/4 cup chopped red onion
- 1/4 cup chopped fresh parsley
- 2 tablespoons olive oil
- 2 tablespoons lemon juice
- 1 teaspoon ground cumin
- Salt and pepper to taste

*Instructions:*

- ✓ In a large bowl, put together the cooked quinoa, chickpeas, diced cucumber, diced red bell pepper, chopped red onion, and chopped fresh parsley.
- ✓ In a small bowl, whisk together olive oil, lemon juice, ground cumin, salt, and pepper.
- ✓ Gently pour the dressing over the salad and toss gently to coat all ingredients.

✓ Chill in the refrigerator for at least 30 minutes before serving to allow flavors to blend.

✓ Serve this refreshing chickpea and quinoa salad as a nutritious meal or side dish!

*Nutritional Information:*

*Calories: 320 | Protein: 12g | Fat: 10g | Carbs: 45g | Fiber: 10g*

# Vegetable Fried Rice

**Servings: 4 | Prep Time: 15 mins | Cooking Time: 15 mins**

*Ingredients:*

- 3 cups cooked rice (most preferably day-old rice)
- 1 cup mixed vegetables (it can be peas, carrots, corn)
- 1/2 cup diced bell peppers
- 1/2 cup diced onion
- 2 cloves garlic, minced
- 2 tablespoons soy sauce
- 1 tablespoon sesame oil
- 2 eggs, beaten (optional)
- Chopped green onions for garnish

*Instructions:*

- ✓ Heat sesame oil in a large skillet or wok over moderate heat.
- ✓ Add minced garlic and diced onion, stir-fry for 1-2 minutes until fragrant.
- ✓ Add the mixed vegetables and diced bell peppers, cook for 3-4 minutes until tender.
- ✓ Push the vegetables to the side of the skillet, pour beaten eggs into the cleared space (if using), and scramble until cooked.
- ✓ Stir in cooked rice and soy sauce, tossing to combine well with the vegetables and eggs.
- ✓ Continue stir-frying for 3-4 minutes until heated through.
- ✓ Garnish with chopped green onions and serve this flavorful vegetable fried rice!

*Nutritional Information:*

*Calories: 280 | Protein: 8g | Fat: 6g | Carbs: 50g | Fiber: 4g*

## Mediterranean Pasta Salad

**Servings: 6 | Prep Time: 15 mins | Cooking Time: 10 mins**

*Ingredients:*

- ● 8 oz pasta (penne or fusilli)
- ● 1 cup cherry tomatoes, halved

- 1/2 cup sliced black olives
- 1/2 cup diced cucumber
- 1/4 cup diced red onion
- 1/4 cup crumbled feta cheese
- 2 tablespoons chopped fresh basil
- 2 tablespoons chopped fresh parsley
- 3 tablespoons olive oil
- 2 tablespoons red wine vinegar
- 1 teaspoon dried oregano
- Salt and pepper to taste

*Instructions:*

✓ Cook pasta in accordance with the package instructions, then drain and rinse with cold water.

✓ In a large bowl, put together the cooked pasta, cherry tomatoes, sliced black olives, diced cucumber, diced red onion, crumbled feta cheese, chopped fresh basil, and chopped fresh parsley.

✓ In a small bowl, whisk together olive oil, red wine vinegar, dried oregano, salt, and pepper.

✓ Gently pour the dressing over the salad and toss gently to coat all ingredients.

✓ Chill in the refrigerator for at least 30 minutes before serving to enhance the flavors.

✓ Serve this vibrant Mediterranean pasta salad as a refreshing dish!

*Nutritional Information:*

*Calories: 260 | Protein: 6g | Fat: 10g | Carbs: 35g | Fiber: 3g*

## Eggplant and Chickpea Curry

**Servings: 4 | Prep Time: 20 mins | Cooking Time: 25 mins**

*Ingredients:*

- 1 large eggplant, diced
- 1 can (15 oz) chickpeas, carefully washed and drained
- 1 onion, finely chopped
- 2 cloves garlic, minced
- 1 can (14 oz) diced tomatoes
- 1 can (14 oz) coconut milk
- 2 tablespoons curry powder
- 1 teaspoon ground cumin
- 1 teaspoon ground coriander
- 1/2 teaspoon turmeric
- 2 tablespoons olive oil
- Salt and pepper to taste
- Chopped cilantro for garnish

- Cooked rice for serving

*Instructions:*

✓ Heat olive oil in a large skillet or pot over moderate heat.

✓ Sauté chopped onion and minced garlic until softened.

✓ Add diced eggplant and cook for 5-7 minutes until slightly tender.

✓ Stir in chickpeas, diced tomatoes, coconut milk, curry powder, ground cumin, ground coriander, turmeric, salt, and pepper.

✓ Simmer for 15-20 minutes until the eggplant is soft and the curry thickens.

✓ Adjust seasoning if needed.

✓ Serve the aromatic eggplant and chickpea curry over cooked rice.

✓ Garnish with chopped cilantro.

*Nutritional Information:*

*Calories: 320 | Protein: 10g | Fat: 15g | Carbs: 45g | Fiber: 12g*

# Caprese Pasta

**Servings: 4 | Prep Time: 10 mins | Cooking Time: 15 mins**

*Ingredients:*

- 8 oz pasta (any pasta of choice such as penne or fusilli)
- 2 cups cherry tomatoes, halved
- 1 cup fresh mozzarella balls, halved
- 1/4 cup fresh basil leaves, torn
- 3 tablespoons olive oil
- 2 tablespoons balsamic vinegar
- Salt and pepper to taste

*Instructions:*

✓ Cook pasta in accordance with the package instructions, then drain and rinse with cold water.

✓ In a large bowl, put together the cooked pasta, halved cherry tomatoes, halved fresh mozzarella balls, and torn fresh basil leaves.

✓ Drizzle olive oil and balsamic vinegar over the salad.

✓ Toss gently to coat all ingredients.

✓ Add a little salt and pepper to your preferred taste.

✓ Serve this delightful Caprese pasta salad as a refreshing dish!

*Nutritional Information:*

*Calories: 320 | Protein: 12g | Fat: 15g | Carbs: 35g | Fiber: 3g*

# Faro and Vegetable Bowl

**Servings: 4 | Prep Time: 15 mins | Cooking Time: 20 mins**

*Ingredients:*

- 1 cup faro, cooked
- 1 cup broccoli florets
- 1 cup diced sweet potatoes
- 1 cup sliced bell peppers (of assorted colors)
- 1/2 cup sliced red onion
- 2 tablespoons olive oil
- 2 tablespoons balsamic vinegar
- 1 teaspoon smoked paprika
- 1/2 teaspoon garlic powder
- Salt and pepper to taste
- Chopped fresh parsley for garnish

*Instructions:*

- ✓ Set the temperature of the oven to 400°F (200°C).
- ✓ On a baking sheet, toss broccoli florets, diced sweet potatoes, sliced bell peppers, and sliced red onion with olive oil, balsamic vinegar, smoked paprika, garlic powder, salt, and pepper.
- ✓ Roast in the oven for fifteen (15) to twenty (20) minutes until vegetables are tender and slightly caramelized.

✓ In a bowl, put together the cooked faro and the roasted vegetables.

✓ Mix well and garnish with chopped fresh parsley before serving this flavorful faro and vegetable bowl!

*Nutritional Information:*

*Calories: 280 | Protein: 6g | Fat: 8g | Carbs: 45g | Fiber: 8g*

# Lentil and Rice Stuffed Bell Peppers

**Servings: 4 | Prep Time: 15 mins | Cooking Time: 40 mins**

*Ingredients:*

- 4 bell peppers, tops removed and seeds carefully removed
- 1 cup cooked brown rice
- 1 cup cooked lentils
- 1 onion, finely chopped
- 2 cloves garlic, minced
- 1 can (14 oz) diced tomatoes
- 1 teaspoon dried oregano
- 1 teaspoon smoked paprika
- Salt and pepper to taste
- Shredded cheese for topping (optional)

◉ Chopped fresh parsley for garnish

*Instructions:*

✓ Set the temperature of the oven to 375°F (190°C).

✓ In a skillet, sauté chopped onion and minced garlic until translucent.

✓ Add cooked brown rice, cooked lentils, diced tomatoes, dried oregano, smoked paprika, salt, and pepper to the skillet. Cook for 5-7 minutes.

✓ Stuff each bell pepper with the lentil and rice mixture.

✓ Place stuffed peppers in a baking dish.

✓ If desired, sprinkle shredded cheese on top of each pepper.

✓ Bake for fifteen (15) to thirty (30) minutes until peppers are tender.

✓ Garnish with chopped fresh parsley before serving these hearty lentil and rice stuffed bell peppers!

*Nutritional Information:*

*Calories: 300 | Protein: 10g | Fat: 5g | Carbs: 50g | Fiber: 12g*

# Spinach and Ricotta Stuffed Shells

**Servings: 4 | Prep Time: 20 mins | Cooking Time: 25 mins**

*Ingredients:*

- 16 jumbo pasta shells, cooked according to package instructions
- 2 cups ricotta cheese
- 1 cup chopped spinach
- 1/2 cup grated Parmesan cheese
- 1 egg, beaten
- 1 teaspoon dried basil
- 1 teaspoon dried oregano
- Salt and pepper to taste
- 2 cups marinara sauce
- Shredded mozzarella cheese for topping

*Instructions:*

- ✓ Set the temperature of the oven to 375°F (190°C).
- ✓ In a bowl, mix the ricotta cheese, chopped spinach, grated Parmesan cheese, beaten egg, dried basil, dried oregano, salt, and pepper.
- ✓ Stuff each cooked pasta shell with the ricotta mixture.
- ✓ Spread marinara sauce in a baking dish.
- ✓ Gently place the stuffed shells in the dish over the sauce.
- ✓ Top with shredded mozzarella cheese.

✓ Bake for 20-25 minutes until the cheese is bubbly and golden.

✓ Serve these delightful spinach and ricotta stuffed shells!

*Nutritional Information:*

*Calories: 350 | Protein: 18g | Fat: 15g | Carbs: 35g | Fiber: 3g*

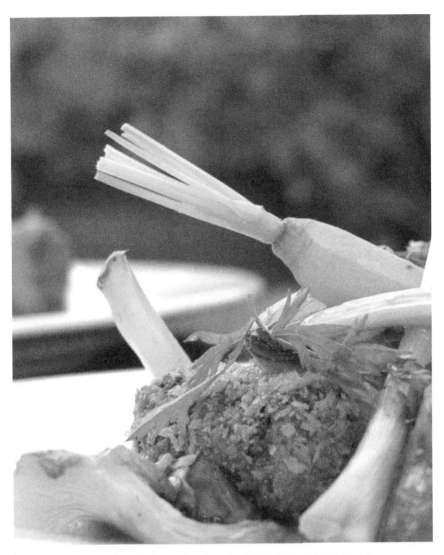

## VEGAN AND VEGETARIAN
## RECIPES

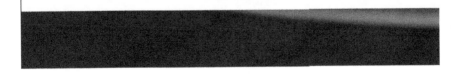

# Quinoa Stuffed Bell Peppers

**Servings: 4 | Prep Time: 20 mins | Cooking Time: 40 mins**

*Ingredients:*

- 4 bell peppers, tops removed and seeds carefully removed
- 1 cup quinoa, cooked
- 1 can (15 oz) black beans, carefully washed and drained
- 1 cup corn kernels
- 1 onion, finely chopped
- 2 cloves garlic, minced
- 1 can (14 oz) diced tomatoes
- 1 teaspoon chili powder
- 1 teaspoon cumin
- 1/2 teaspoon paprika
- Salt and pepper to taste
- Chopped fresh cilantro for garnish
- Avocado slices for serving (optional)

*Instructions:*

- ✓ Set the temperature of the oven to 375°F (190°C).
- ✓ In a skillet, sauté chopped onion and minced garlic until softened.

✓ Add cooked quinoa, black beans, corn kernels, diced tomatoes, chili powder, cumin, paprika, salt, and pepper to the skillet. Cook for 5-7 minutes.

✓ Stuff each bell pepper with the quinoa and vegetable mixture.

✓ Place stuffed peppers in a baking dish.

✓ Cover with foil and bake for thirty (30) minutes.

✓ Remove the foil and bake for an additional 10 minutes until peppers are tender and slightly browned.

✓ Garnish with chopped fresh cilantro.

✓ Serve these delicious quinoa stuffed bell peppers with avocado slices if desired!

*Nutritional Information:*

*Calories: 320 | Protein: 15g | Fat: 5g | Carbs: 60g | Fiber: 12g*

# Vegan Lentil Soup

**Servings: 6 | Prep Time: 15 mins | Cooking Time: 30 mins**

*Ingredients:*

- 1 cup dried green lentils
- 1 onion, finely chopped
- 2 carrots, diced
- 2 celery stalks, diced

- 2 cloves garlic, minced
- 1 can (14 oz) diced tomatoes
- 6 cups vegetable broth
- 1 teaspoon ground cumin
- 1 teaspoon smoked paprika
- 1 teaspoon dried thyme
- Salt and pepper to taste
- Chopped fresh parsley for garnish

*Instructions:*

✓ Rinse dried green lentils under cold water and set aside.

✓ In a large pot, sauté chopped onion, diced carrots, diced celery, and minced garlic until softened.

✓ Add diced tomatoes, vegetable broth, dried green lentils, ground cumin, smoked paprika, dried thyme, salt, and pepper to the pot.

✓ Bring to a boil, then reduce heat and simmer for 25-30 minutes until lentils are tender.

✓ Adjust seasoning if needed.

✓ Serve this comforting vegan lentil soup hot, garnished with chopped fresh parsley.

*Nutritional Information:*

*Calories: 240 | Protein: 15g | Fat: 2g | Carbs: 40g | Fiber: 15g*

# Eggplant Parmesan

**Servings: 4 | Prep Time: 25 mins | Cooking Time: 45 mins**

*Ingredients:*

- 2 medium eggplants, sliced into rounds
- 1 cup breadcrumbs (use vegan breadcrumbs if desired)
- 1 cup marinara sauce
- 1/2 cup vegan Parmesan cheese
- 1/2 cup vegan mozzarella cheese
- 2 tablespoons olive oil
- 1 teaspoon dried oregano
- Salt and pepper to taste
- Chopped fresh basil for garnish

*Instructions:*

- ✓ Set the temperature of the oven to 375°F (190°C).
- ✓ Dip eggplant slices in olive oil, then coat them in breadcrumbs.
- ✓ Place the coated eggplant slices on a baking sheet lined with parchment paper.
- ✓ Bake for 20-25 minutes until eggplant slices are tender and golden.
- ✓ In a baking dish, spread a layer of marinara sauce.
- ✓ Place half of the baked eggplant slices on top of the sauce.

- ✓ Sprinkle with vegan Parmesan cheese and vegan mozzarella cheese.
- ✓ Add another layer of marinara sauce and the remaining eggplant slices.
- ✓ Sprinkle with more vegan cheeses, dried oregano, salt, and pepper.
- ✓ Bake for 20 minutes until the cheese is melted and bubbly.
- ✓ Garnish with chopped fresh basil before serving this delectable eggplant Parmesan!

*Nutritional Information:*

*Calories: 280 | Protein: 10g | Fat: 10g | Carbs: 35g | Fiber: 8g*

# Vegan Cauliflower Curry

**Servings: 4 | Prep Time: 15 mins | Cooking Time: 25 mins**

*Ingredients:*

- 1 medium cauliflower, cut into florets
- 1 onion, finely chopped
- 2 cloves garlic, minced
- 1 can (14 oz) coconut milk
- 1 can (14 oz) diced tomatoes
- 2 tablespoons curry powder

- 1 teaspoon ground cumin
- 1 teaspoon turmeric
- 1 teaspoon paprika
- 2 tablespoons olive oil
- Salt and pepper to taste
- Chopped fresh cilantro for garnish
- Cooked rice for serving

## Instructions:

✓ Heat olive oil in a large skillet or pot over moderate heat.

✓ Sauté chopped onion and minced garlic until softened.

✓ Add cauliflower florets and cook for 5-7 minutes until slightly tender.

✓ Stir in diced tomatoes, coconut milk, curry powder, ground cumin, turmeric, paprika, salt, and pepper.

✓ Simmer for 15-20 minutes until cauliflower is cooked through and the curry thickens.

✓ Adjust seasoning if needed.

✓ Serve the aromatic vegan cauliflower curry over cooked rice.

✓ Garnish with chopped fresh cilantro.

## Nutritional Information:

*Calories: 290 | Protein: 6g | Fat: 15g | Carbs: 35g | Fiber: 10g*

# Sweet Potato and Black Bean Enchiladas

**Servings: 4 | Prep Time: 25 mins | Cooking Time: 30 mins**

*Ingredients:*

- 8 corn tortillas
- 2 cups cooked sweet potatoes, mashed
- 1 can (15 oz) black beans, carefully washed and drained
- 1 red bell pepper, diced
- 1 onion, finely chopped
- 2 cloves garlic, minced
- 1 can (14 oz) enchilada sauce
- 1 teaspoon cumin
- 1 teaspoon chili powder
- Salt and pepper to taste
- Chopped fresh cilantro for garnish
- Sliced avocado for topping (optional)

*Instructions:*

- ✓ Set the temperature of the oven to 375°F (190°C).
- ✓ In a skillet, sauté chopped onion and minced garlic until softened.
- ✓ Add diced red bell pepper and cook for 3-4 minutes until tender.

✓ Stir in mashed sweet potatoes, black beans, cumin, chili powder, salt, and pepper. Mix well.

✓ Warm the corn tortillas slightly to make them pliable.

✓ Spoon the sweet potato and black bean mixture onto each tortilla and roll them up.

✓ Place the rolled tortillas seam-side down in a baking dish.

✓ Pour enchilada sauce over the top of the rolled tortillas.

✓ Bake for 20-25 minutes until the sauce is bubbly.

✓ Garnish with chopped fresh cilantro and serve these flavorful sweet potato and black bean enchiladas.

✓ Top with sliced avocado if desired!

*Nutritional Information:*

*Calories: 320 | Protein: 10g | Fat: 5g | Carbs: 60g | Fiber: 12g*

## Vegan Mushroom Stroganoff

**Servings: 4 | Prep Time: 15 mins | Cooking Time: 25 mins**

*Ingredients:*

- 8 oz fettuccine pasta
- 2 cups sliced mushrooms
- 1 onion, finely chopped
- 2 cloves garlic, minced

- 1 can (14 oz) coconut milk
- 2 tablespoons flour (use cornstarch for gluten-free)
- 2 tablespoons nutritional yeast
- 1 tablespoon soy sauce
- 1 teaspoon paprika
- Salt and pepper to taste
- Chopped fresh parsley for garnish

*Instructions:*

- ✓ Cook the fettuccine pasta in accordance with the package instructions, then drain and set aside.
- ✓ In a skillet, sauté chopped onion and minced garlic until translucent.
- ✓ Add sliced mushrooms and cook for 5-7 minutes until they release their juices.
- ✓ In a bowl, whisk together coconut milk, flour (or cornstarch), nutritional yeast, soy sauce, paprika, salt, and pepper.
- ✓ Pour the coconut milk mixture into the skillet with the mushrooms.
- ✓ Stir well and simmer for 10-12 minutes until the sauce thickens.
- ✓ Adjust seasoning if needed.
- ✓ Serve the creamy vegan mushroom stroganoff over cooked fettuccine.
- ✓ Garnish with chopped fresh parsley.

*Nutritional Information:*

*Calories: 380 | Protein: 10g | Fat: 15g | Carbs: 50g | Fiber: 6g*

# Vegan Lentil Sloppy Joes

**Servings: 4 | Prep Time: 15 mins | Cooking Time: 25 mins**

*Ingredients:*

- 1 cup dry lentils
- 1 onion, finely chopped
- 2 cloves garlic, minced
- 1 bell pepper, diced
- 1 can (14 oz) diced tomatoes
- 1/4 cup tomato paste
- 2 tablespoons maple syrup
- 2 tablespoons apple cider vinegar
- 1 tablespoon Dijon mustard
- 1 teaspoon chili powder
- 1 teaspoon smoked paprika
- Salt and pepper to taste
- Hamburger buns or bread of choice

*Instructions:*

✓ Rinse dry lentils under cold water and cook in accordance with the package instructions. Drain and set aside.

✓ In a skillet, sauté chopped onion and minced garlic until translucent.

✓ Add diced bell pepper and cook for 3-4 minutes until softened.

✓ Stir in cooked lentils, diced tomatoes, tomato paste, maple syrup, apple cider vinegar, Dijon mustard, chili powder, smoked paprika, salt, and pepper.

✓ Simmer for fifteen (15) to twenty (20) minutes until the flavors meld together and the mixture thickens.

✓ Adjust seasoning if needed.

✓ Serve the flavorful vegan lentil sloppy joe mixture on hamburger buns or bread slices.

*Nutritional Information:*

*Calories: 320 | Protein: 15g | Fat: 2g | Carbs: 60g | Fiber: 15g*

# Vegan Chickpea Curry

**Servings: 4 | Prep Time: 15 mins | Cooking Time: 25 mins**

*Ingredients:*

● 2 cans (15 oz each) chickpeas, carefully washed and drained

- 1 onion, finely chopped
- 2 cloves garlic, minced
- 1 bell pepper, diced
- 1 can (14 oz) coconut milk
- 1 can (14 oz) diced tomatoes
- 2 tablespoons curry powder
- 1 teaspoon ground cumin
- 1 teaspoon ground coriander
- 1/2 teaspoon turmeric
- 2 tablespoons olive oil
- Salt and pepper to taste
- Chopped fresh cilantro for garnish
- Cooked rice for serving

*Instructions:*

✓ Heat olive oil in a large skillet or pot over moderate heat.

✓ Sauté chopped onion and minced garlic until softened.

✓ Add diced bell pepper and cook for 3-4 minutes until tender.

✓ Stir in drained and rinsed chickpeas, diced tomatoes, coconut milk, curry powder, ground cumin, ground coriander, turmeric, salt, and pepper.

✓ Simmer for fifteen (15) to twenty (20) minutes until flavors meld together and the curry thickens.

✓ Adjust seasoning if needed.

✓ Serve the aromatic vegan chickpea curry over cooked rice.

✓ Garnish with chopped fresh cilantro.

*Nutritional Information:*

*Calories: 350 | Protein: 15g | Fat: 10g | Carbs: 45g | Fiber: 12g*

# Vegan Lentil Meatballs

**Servings: 4 | Prep Time: 20 mins | Cooking Time: 25 mins**

*Ingredients:*

- 1 cup cooked lentils
- 1 onion, finely chopped
- 2 cloves garlic, minced
- 1 cup breadcrumbs (use vegan breadcrumbs if desired)
- 2 tablespoons tomato paste
- 2 tablespoons ground flaxseeds
- 2 tablespoons chopped fresh parsley
- 1 teaspoon dried oregano
- Salt and pepper to taste
- 2 tablespoons olive oil

*Instructions:*

- ✓ Set the temperature of the oven to 375°F (190°C) and line a baking sheet with parchment paper.
- ✓ In a bowl, mash the cooked lentils slightly.
- ✓ In a skillet, sauté the chopped onion and minced garlic until softened.
- ✓ In the bowl with mashed the lentils, add sautéed onion and garlic, breadcrumbs, tomato paste, ground flaxseeds, chopped fresh parsley, dried oregano, salt, and pepper. Mix until well combined.
- ✓ Shape the mixture into meatballs and place them on the prepared baking sheet.
- ✓ Drizzle olive oil over the meatballs.
- ✓ Bake for twenty (20) to twenty-five (25) minutes until golden and cooked through.
- ✓ Serve these flavorful vegan lentil meatballs with your favorite sauce or pasta!

*Nutritional Information:*

*Calories: 220 | Protein: 10g | Fat: 8g | Carbs: 30g | Fiber: 8g*

# Vegan Butternut Squash Soup

**Servings: 4 | Prep Time: 15 mins | Cooking Time: 35 mins**

*Ingredients:*

- 1 butternut squash, peeled and diced
- 1 onion, finely chopped
- 2 carrots, diced
- 2 cloves garlic, minced
- 4 cups vegetable broth
- 1 can (14 oz) coconut milk
- 1 tablespoon olive oil
- 1 teaspoon ground cumin
- 1 teaspoon curry powder
- Salt and pepper to taste
- Roasted pumpkin seeds for garnish

*Instructions:*

- ✓ Heat olive oil in a large pot over moderate heat.
- ✓ Sauté chopped onion and minced garlic until translucent.
- ✓ Add diced butternut squash and carrots, cook for 5-7 minutes until slightly softened.
- ✓ Stir in vegetable broth, coconut milk, ground cumin, curry powder, salt, and pepper.

✓ Bring to a boil, then reduce heat and simmer for twenty (20) to twenty-five (25) minutes until vegetables are tender.

✓ Use an immersion blender or gently transfer the soup to a blender to puree until everything is smooth.

✓ Adjust seasoning if needed.

✓ Serve this creamy vegan butternut squash soup topped with roasted pumpkin seeds.

*Nutritional Information:*

*Calories: 250 | Protein: 5g | Fat: 15g | Carbs: 25g | Fiber: 5g*

# Vegan Chili

**Servings: 6 | Prep Time: 15 mins | Cooking Time: 35 mins**

*Ingredients:*

- 2 cans (15 oz each) kidney beans, carefully washed and drained
- 1 can (14 oz) diced tomatoes
- 1 onion, finely chopped
- 2 cloves garlic, minced
- 1 bell pepper, diced
- 1 cup corn kernels
- 2 tablespoons tomato paste
- 2 tablespoons chili powder

- 1 teaspoon cumin
- 1 teaspoon paprika
- 1 tablespoon olive oil
- Salt and pepper to taste
- Chopped fresh cilantro for garnish
- Vegan sour cream for topping (optional)

## Instructions:

- ✓ Heat olive oil in a large pot over moderate heat.
- ✓ Sauté chopped onion and minced garlic until softened.
- ✓ Add diced bell pepper and cook for 3-4 minutes until tender.
- ✓ Stir in drained and rinsed kidney beans, diced tomatoes, corn kernels, tomato paste, chili powder, cumin, paprika, salt, and pepper.
- ✓ Simmer for twenty (20) to twenty-five (25) minutes until flavors meld together and the chili thickens.
- ✓ Adjust seasoning if needed.
- ✓ Serve the hearty vegan chili hot, garnished with chopped fresh cilantro.
- ✓ Top with vegan sour cream if desired!

## Nutritional Information:

*Calories: 280 | Protein: 12g | Fat: 5g | Carbs: 50g | Fiber: 15g*

## Vegan Cauliflower Buffalo Wings

**Servings: 4 | Prep Time: 15 mins | Cooking Time: 25 mins**

*Ingredients:*

- 1 head cauliflower, cut into florets
- 1 cup flour (use chickpea flour for gluten-free)
- 1 cup plant-based milk (it can be almond milk)
- 1 teaspoon garlic powder
- 1 teaspoon onion powder
- 1/2 teaspoon paprika
- 1 cup buffalo sauce (vegan-friendly)
- 2 tablespoons olive oil
- Salt and pepper to taste
- Vegan ranch or blue cheese dressing for dipping (optional)

*Instructions:*

- ✓ Preheat the oven to 450°F (230°C) and line a baking sheet with parchment paper.
- ✓ In a bowl, whisk together flour, plant-based milk, garlic powder, onion powder, paprika, salt, and pepper to make a batter.
- ✓ Dip each cauliflower floret into the batter, coating evenly, and place them on the prepared baking sheet.
- ✓ Bake for twenty (20) minutes until the cauliflower is slightly crispy.

✓ In a separate bowl, put together the buffalo sauce and olive oil.

✓ Remove cauliflower from the oven and toss in the buffalo sauce mixture until coated.

✓ Place back on the baking sheet and bake for an additional 5 minutes.

✓ Serve these delicious vegan cauliflower buffalo wings with vegan ranch or blue cheese dressing for dipping!

*Nutritional Information:*

*Calories: 180 | Protein: 5g | Fat: 7g | Carbs: 25g | Fiber: 5g*

# Vegan Black Bean Burgers

**Servings: 4 | Prep Time: 20 mins | Cooking Time: 15 mins**

*Ingredients:*

- 1 can (15 oz) black beans, carefully washed and drained
- 1/2 cup breadcrumbs (use gluten-free if needed)
- 1/4 cup finely chopped onion
- 2 cloves garlic, minced
- 1 teaspoon ground cumin
- 1 teaspoon smoked paprika
- Salt and pepper to taste
- 2 tablespoons olive oil

- Burger buns and toppings of choice (lettuce, tomato, avocado, etc.)

*Instructions:*

✓ In a bowl, mash the black beans with a fork or potato masher.

✓ Add breadcrumbs, finely chopped onion, minced garlic, ground cumin, smoked paprika, salt, and pepper. Mix until well combined.

✓ Divide the mixture into four portions and shape them into burger patties.

✓ Heat olive oil in a skillet over moderate heat.

✓ Cook the burger patties for 3-4 minutes on each side until golden brown and heated through.

✓ Toast burger buns if desired and assemble the black bean burgers with your favorite toppings.

*Nutritional Information:*

*Calories: 250 | Protein: 10g | Fat: 8g | Carbs: 35g | Fiber: 10g*

# Vegan Chickpea Salad Sandwich

**Servings: 2 | Prep Time: 10 mins | Cooking Time: 0 min**

*Ingredients:*

- 1 can (15 oz) chickpeas, carefully washed and drained
- 2 tablespoons vegan mayonnaise
- 1 tablespoon Dijon mustard
- 2 tablespoons chopped celery
- 2 tablespoons chopped red onion
- 2 tablespoons chopped fresh parsley
- Salt and pepper to taste
- Bread slices for sandwich
- Lettuce leaves and tomato slices for topping

*Instructions:*

- ✓ In a bowl, mash the chickpeas with a fork or potato masher.
- ✓ Add vegan mayonnaise, Dijon mustard, chopped celery, chopped red onion, chopped fresh parsley, salt, and pepper. Mix until everything is well combined.
- ✓ Spread the chickpea salad onto bread slices.
- ✓ Top with lettuce leaves, tomato slices, and another bread slice to make a sandwich.

*Nutritional Information:*

*Calories: 280 | Protein: 10g | Fat: 10g | Carbs: 35g | Fiber: 10g*

# Vegan Tofu Stir-Fry

**Servings: 4 | Prep Time: 15 mins | Cooking Time: 15 mins**

*Ingredients:*

- 14 oz firm tofu, gently pressed and nicely cubed
- 2 cups mixed vegetables (it can be bell peppers, broccoli, carrots, snap peas, etc.), chopped
- 1 onion, thinly sliced
- 2 cloves garlic, minced
- 1/4 cup soy sauce or tamari
- 2 tablespoons maple syrup or agave nectar
- 1 tablespoon sesame oil
- 1 tablespoon cornstarch
- 2 tablespoons water
- Cooked rice or quinoa for serving
- Sesame seeds and chopped green onions for garnish

*Instructions:*

- ✓ In a bowl, mix the soy sauce or tamari, maple syrup or agave nectar, sesame oil, cornstarch, and water to make the sauce. Set aside.
- ✓ Heat a skillet or wok over moderate to high heat.
- ✓ Add cubed tofu and cook until golden brown on all sides. Remove from the skillet and set aside.

✓ In the same skillet, add a bit of oil if needed, and sauté sliced onion and minced garlic until fragrant.

✓ Add chopped mixed vegetables and stir-fry for 4-5 minutes until tender-crisp.

✓ Return the cooked tofu to the skillet and pour the sauce over the tofu and vegetables.

✓ Stir-fry for another 2-3 minutes until everything is coated in the sauce and heated through.

✓ Serve this delicious vegan tofu stir-fry over cooked rice or quinoa.

✓ Nicely garnish with sesame seeds and chopped green onions.

*Nutritional Information:*

*Calories: 280 | Protein: 15g | Fat: 10g | Carbs: 35g | Fiber: 8g*

# Vegan Zucchini Noodles with Pesto

**Servings: 2 | Prep Time: 15 mins | Cooking Time: 0 min**

*Ingredients:*

⊙ 2 medium zucchinis, spiralized into noodles

⊙ 1/2 cup fresh basil leaves

⊙ 1/4 cup pine nuts

⊙ 2 tablespoons nutritional yeast

- 2 tablespoons olive oil
- 1 clove garlic
- Salt and pepper to taste
- Cherry tomatoes for garnish (optional)

## Instructions:

✓ In a food processor, put together the fresh basil leaves, pine nuts, nutritional yeast, olive oil, garlic, salt, and pepper. Blend until smooth to make the pesto sauce.

✓ In a skillet, heat a bit of olive oil over moderate heat.

✓ Add zucchini noodles and sauté for 2-3 minutes until slightly softened.

✓ Add the prepared pesto sauce to the skillet and toss the noodles until well coated and heated through.

✓ Serve the vegan zucchini noodles with pesto and garnish with cherry tomatoes if desired.

## Nutritional Information:

*Calories: 200 | Protein: 6g | Fat: 15g | Carbs: 10g | Fiber: 4g*

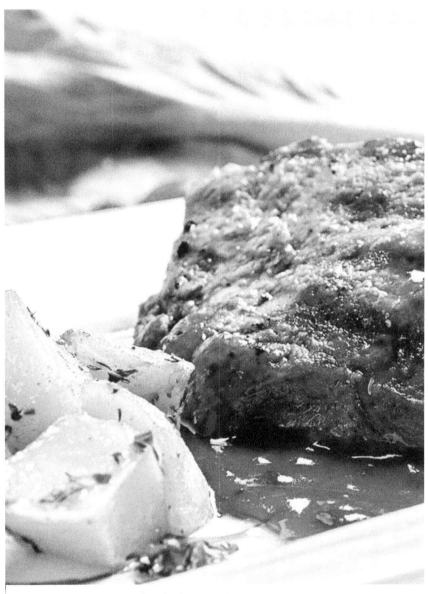

# POULTRY AND MEAT RECIPES

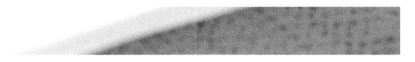

# Classic Roast Chicken

**Servings: 4 | Prep Time: 15 mins | Cooking Time: 120 mins**

*Ingredients:*

- 1 whole chicken (about 4 lbs.)
- 4 tablespoons butter, softened
- 2 cloves garlic, minced
- 1 lemon, halved
- Fresh rosemary sprigs
- Salt and pepper to taste
- Olive oil

*Instructions:*

- ✓ Set the temperature of the oven to 425°F (220°C).
- ✓ Rinse the chicken and pat dry with paper towels.
- ✓ In a small bowl, put together the softened butter with minced garlic.
- ✓ Carefully lift the skin of the chicken and rub the garlic butter underneath the skin and all over the chicken.
- ✓ Season the chicken cavity with salt and pepper. Stuff it with lemon halves and a few sprigs of fresh rosemary.
- ✓ Gently tie the legs together with kitchen twine.
- ✓ Drizzle olive oil over the chicken and rub it all over the skin. Season with salt and pepper.

- ✓ Gently put the chicken on a rack in a roasting pan breast-side up.
- ✓ Roast for about 1 hour 30 minutes or until the internal temperature reaches 165°F (74°C) in the thickest part of the thigh.
- ✓ Let the chicken rest for 10-15 minutes before carving.
- ✓ Carve and serve this classic roast chicken with your favorite sides!

*Nutritional Information:*

*Calories: 350 | Protein: 30g | Fat: 25g | Carbs: 1g | Fiber: 0g*

# Beef Stroganoff

**Servings: 4 | Prep Time: 15 mins | Cooking Time: 30 mins**

*Ingredients:*

- 1 lb. beef sirloin or tenderloin, thinly and carefully sliced
- 1 onion, thinly sliced
- 2 cloves garlic, minced
- 8 oz mushrooms, sliced
- 2 tablespoons butter
- 2 tablespoons all-purpose flour
- 1 cup beef broth
- 1 tablespoon Dijon mustard

- 1/2 cup sour cream
- Salt and pepper to taste
- Chopped fresh parsley for garnish
- Cooked egg noodles or rice for serving

*Instructions:*

✓ Heat a skillet over moderate to high heat and melt butter.

✓ Add thinly sliced beef and cook until browned. Carefully remove beef from the skillet and put it aside.

✓ In the same skillet, sauté thinly sliced onion until softened.

✓ Add minced garlic and sliced mushrooms. Cook until mushrooms are golden brown.

✓ Sprinkle flour over the mushrooms and onions. Stir and cook for 1-2 minutes.

✓ Slowly pour in beef broth while stirring continuously to avoid lumps.

✓ Stir in Dijon mustard and let the sauce simmer for 5 minutes until thickened.

✓ Return the cooked beef to the skillet and mix well with the sauce.

✓ Turn off the heat and stir in sour cream. Season with salt and pepper.

✓ Serve this comforting beef stroganoff over cooked egg noodles or rice.

✓ Garnish with chopped fresh parsley.

*Nutritional Information:*

*Calories: 380 | Protein: 30g | Fat: 20g | Carbs: 15g | Fiber: 2g*

## Grilled Lemon Herb Chicken

**Servings: 4 | Prep Time: 10 mins | Cooking Time: 15 mins**

*Ingredients:*

- 4 boneless, skinless chicken breasts
- Zest and juice of 1 lemon
- 2 tablespoons olive oil
- 2 cloves garlic, minced
- 1 teaspoon dried thyme
- 1 teaspoon dried rosemary
- Salt and pepper to taste
- Lemon wedges for serving
- Fresh parsley for garnish

*Instructions:*

✓ In a bowl, put together the lemon zest, lemon juice, olive oil, minced garlic, dried thyme, dried rosemary, salt, and pepper.

✓ Place chicken breasts in a resealable plastic bag or shallow dish and pour the marinade over them. Marinate for at least 30 minutes.

✓ Preheat the grill to moderate to high heat.

✓ Remove chicken from the marinade and discard excess marinade.

✓ Grill chicken for about six (6) to seven (7) minutes on each side or until cooked through with grill marks.

✓ Remove from the grill and let the chicken rest for a few minutes.

✓ Serve this flavorful grilled lemon herb chicken with lemon wedges and garnish with fresh parsley.

*Nutritional Information:*

*Calories: 280 | Protein: 35g | Fat: 12g | Carbs: 2g | Fiber: 0g*

# Pork Tenderloin with Apple Glaze

**Servings: 4 | Prep Time: 15 mins | Cooking Time: 25 mins**

*Ingredients:*

- 1 lb. pork tenderloin
- 2 apples, peeled and sliced
- 2 tablespoons olive oil
- 2 tablespoons honey

- 2 tablespoons Dijon mustard
- 2 tablespoons apple cider vinegar
- Salt and pepper to taste
- Fresh thyme for garnish

*Instructions:*

✓ Set the temperature of the oven to 400°F (200°C).

✓ Season pork tenderloin with salt and pepper.

✓ Heat olive oil in an oven-proof skillet over moderate to high heat.

✓ Gently sear the pork tenderloin on all sides until browned.

✓ Remove the skillet from heat and place apple slices around the pork tenderloin.

✓ In a bowl, put together the honey, Dijon mustard, and apple cider vinegar. Pour the mixture over the pork and apples.

✓ Transfer the skillet to the preheated oven and roast for 20-25 minutes or until the internal temperature of the pork reaches 145°F (63°C).

✓ Let the pork rest for a few minutes before slicing.

✓ Serve this succulent pork tenderloin with apple glaze and garnish with fresh thyme.

*Nutritional Information:*

Calories: 280 | Protein: 25g | Fat: 10g | Carbs: 20g | Fiber: 3g

# Chicken Piccata

**Servings: 4 | Prep Time: 15 mins | Cooking Time: 20 mins**

*Ingredients:*

- 4 boneless, skinless chicken breasts
- Salt and pepper to taste
- 1/2 cup all-purpose flour
- 2 tablespoons olive oil
- 4 tablespoons unsalted butter
- 1/2 cup chicken broth
- 1/4 cup fresh lemon juice
- 1/4 cup capers, drained
- 2 tablespoons chopped fresh parsley

*Instructions:*

- ✓ Place chicken breasts between plastic wrap and pound them to an even thickness. Adjust with a little salt and pepper to your preferred taste.
- ✓ Gently dredge the chicken breasts in the flour, and shake off the excess.
- ✓ Heat olive oil in a skillet over moderate to high heat.

✓ Cook chicken breasts for 4-5 minutes on each side until golden brown and cooked through. Gently remove from the skillet and put it aside.

✓ In the same skillet, melt butter. Add chicken broth, lemon juice, and capers. Simmer for two (2) to three (3) minutes to reduce slightly.

✓ Return the chicken breasts to the skillet and cook for an additional two (2) minutes, spooning the sauce over them.

✓ Sprinkle chopped fresh parsley over the chicken piccata.

✓ Serve the flavorful chicken piccata with the tangy sauce.

*Nutritional Information:*

*Calories: 320 | Protein: 30g | Fat: 18g | Carbs: 10g | Fiber: 1g*

# Honey Garlic Glazed Salmon

**Servings: 4 | Prep Time: 10 mins | Cooking Time: 15 mins**

*Ingredients:*

- 4 salmon filets
- Salt and pepper to taste
- 4 tablespoons honey
- 3 tablespoons soy sauce
- 2 cloves garlic, minced

- 1 tablespoon olive oil
- 1 tablespoon chopped fresh parsley
- Lemon wedges for serving

*Instructions:*

✓ Adjust the salmon filets with a little salt and pepper.

✓ In a bowl, put together the honey, soy sauce, and minced garlic to make the glaze.

✓ Heat olive oil in a skillet over moderate to high heat.

✓ Gently put the salmon filets in the skillet and cook for 3-4 minutes on each side until browned and cooked to desired doneness.

✓ Pour the honey garlic glaze over the salmon filets in the skillet.

✓ Allow the glaze to thicken for 1-2 minutes, continuously spooning it over the salmon.

✓ Sprinkle chopped fresh parsley over the glazed salmon.

✓ Serve the honey garlic glazed salmon with lemon wedges.

*Nutritional Information:*

*Calories: 320 | Protein: 25g | Fat: 18g | Carbs: 15g | Fiber: 0g*

# Turkey Meatballs in Marinara Sauce

**Servings: 4 | Prep Time: 20 mins | Cooking Time: 25 mins**

*Ingredients:*

## For the meatballs:

- 1 lb. ground turkey
- 1/2 cup breadcrumbs
- 1/4 cup grated Parmesan cheese
- 1 egg
- 2 cloves garlic, minced
- 2 tablespoons chopped fresh parsley
- Salt and pepper to taste

## For the marinara sauce:

- 2 cups marinara sauce
- 1 tablespoon olive oil
- 1/2 onion, finely chopped
- 2 cloves garlic, minced
- 1 teaspoon dried oregano
- 1 teaspoon dried basil
- Salt and pepper to taste
- Chopped fresh basil for garnish

## *Instructions:*

✓ Set the temperature of the oven to 400°F (200°C).

✓ In a bowl, put together the ground turkey, breadcrumbs, grated Parmesan cheese, egg, minced garlic, chopped parsley, salt, and pepper. Form into meatballs.

✓ Place meatballs on a baking sheet lined with parchment paper and bake for 15-18 minutes until cooked through.

✓ Meanwhile, heat olive oil in a saucepan over moderate heat. Sauté chopped onion and minced garlic until everything is softened.

✓ Add marinara sauce, dried oregano, dried basil, salt, and pepper to the saucepan. Simmer for 5-7 minutes.

✓ Add the cooked meatballs to the marinara sauce and simmer for an additional 5 minutes.

✓ Serve the turkey meatballs in marinara sauce, garnished with chopped fresh basil.

*Nutritional Information:*

*Calories: 280 | Protein: 25g | Fat: 12g | Carbs: 18g | Fiber: 2g*

# Beef and Broccoli Stir-Fry

**Servings: 4 | Prep Time: 15 mins | Cooking Time: 15 mins**

*Ingredients:*

- 1 lb. flank steak, thinly sliced
- 3 cups broccoli florets
- 1/4 cup soy sauce
- 2 tablespoons brown sugar
- 2 tablespoons oyster sauce
- 1 tablespoon sesame oil
- 3 cloves garlic, minced
- 1 teaspoon grated ginger
- 2 tablespoons cornstarch
- 2 tablespoons water
- Cooked rice for serving

*Instructions:*

- ✓ In a bowl, put together the soy sauce, brown sugar, oyster sauce, sesame oil, minced garlic, and grated ginger.
- ✓ In another bowl, put together the cornstarch and water to create a slurry.
- ✓ Heat a skillet or wok over high heat. Add a bit of oil.
- ✓ Stir-fry thinly sliced flank steak until browned. Gently remove from the skillet and put it aside.

✓ Stir-fry broccoli florets in the same skillet until tender-crisp.

✓ Return the cooked beef to the skillet with broccoli.

✓ Pour the soy sauce mixture over the beef and broccoli. Stir well.

✓ Add the cornstarch slurry and cook for a few minutes until the sauce thickens.

✓ Serve this delicious beef and broccoli stir-fry over cooked rice.

*Nutritional Information:*

*Calories: 320 | Protein: 30g | Fat: 10g | Carbs: 25g | Fiber: 4g*

# Lemon Garlic Butter Shrimp

**Servings: 4 | Prep Time: 10 mins | Cooking Time: 10 mins**

*Ingredients:*

- 1 lb. large shrimp, peeled and veins removed
- Salt and pepper to taste
- 2 tablespoons olive oil
- 4 tablespoons unsalted butter
- 4 cloves garlic, minced
- Zest and juice of 1 lemon
- 2 tablespoons chopped fresh parsley

*Instructions:*

✓ Pat the shrimp dry with paper towels. Adjust with a little salt and pepper to your preferred taste.

✓ Heat olive oil in a skillet over moderate to high heat.

✓ Add shrimp to the skillet and cook for 2-3 minutes on each side until pink and opaque. Gently remove from the skillet and put it aside.

✓ In the same skillet, melt butter. Add minced garlic and cook for one to two minutes until fragrant.

✓ Stir in lemon zest and lemon juice. Bring to a simmer.

✓ Return the cooked shrimp to the skillet and toss in the lemon garlic butter sauce.

✓ Cook for an additional minute until heated through and coated in the sauce.

✓ Garnish with chopped fresh parsley.

✓ Serve the flavorful lemon garlic butter shrimp immediately.

*Nutritional Information:*

*Calories: 220 | Protein: 25g | Fat: 12g | Carbs: 2g | Fiber: 0g*

# Stuffed Bell Peppers with Ground Turkey

**Servings: 4 | Prep Time: 20 mins | Cooking Time: 45 mins**

*Ingredients:*

- 4 bell peppers, halved and seeds carefully removed
- 1 lb. ground turkey
- 1 cup cooked quinoa
- 1 onion, diced
- 2 cloves garlic, minced
- 1 can (14 oz) diced tomatoes, drained
- 1 cup shredded mozzarella cheese
- 1 teaspoon dried oregano
- 1 teaspoon dried basil
- Salt and pepper to taste
- Chopped fresh parsley for garnish

*Instructions:*

- ✓ Set the temperature of the oven to 375°F (190°C).
- ✓ Place halved bell peppers in a baking dish.
- ✓ In a skillet, cook ground turkey until browned. Drain excess fat.
- ✓ Add diced onion and minced garlic to the skillet. Cook until onion is softened.

✓ Stir in cooked quinoa, diced tomatoes, shredded mozzarella cheese, dried oregano, dried basil, salt, and pepper. Mix well.

✓ Spoon the turkey and quinoa mixture into each bell pepper half.

✓ Cover the baking dish with foil and bake for 35-40 minutes until bell peppers are tender.

✓ Remove the foil and bake for an additional 5 minutes to melt the cheese.

✓ Neatly garnish with chopped fresh parsley before serving.

*Nutritional Information:*

*Calories: 320 | Protein: 25g | Fat: 10g | Carbs: 30g | Fiber: 6g*

# Teriyaki Chicken Skewers

**Servings: 4 | Prep Time: 15 mins | Cooking Time: 15 mins**

*Ingredients:*

- 1 lb. boneless, skinless chicken thighs, cut them into smaller chunks

- 1/2 cup soy sauce

- 1/4 cup brown sugar

- 2 tablespoons rice vinegar

- 2 cloves garlic, minced

- 1 tablespoon grated ginger

- 1 tablespoon cornstarch
- 1 tablespoon water
- Sesame seeds and chopped green onions (used for garnishing)

*Instructions:*

✓ In a bowl, put together the soy sauce, brown sugar, rice vinegar, minced garlic, and grated ginger.

✓ Thread chicken chunks onto skewers.

✓ Grill or cook the chicken skewers on a grill pan over medium-high heat for about 6-8 minutes on each side until cooked through.

✓ Meanwhile, in a saucepan, bring the soy sauce mixture to a simmer.

✓ In a small bowl, put together the cornstarch and water to create a slurry. Gently stir the slurry into the simmering sauce until everything is thickened.

✓ Brush the teriyaki sauce over the chicken skewers.

✓ Serve these delightful teriyaki chicken skewers sprinkled with sesame seeds and chopped green onions.

*Nutritional Information:*

*Calories: 280 | Protein: 25g | Fat: 8g | Carbs: 25g | Fiber: 1g*

# BBQ Pulled Pork Sandwiches

**Servings: 4 | Prep Time: 10 mins | Cooking Time: 6 hours**

*Ingredients:*

- 2 lbs. pork shoulder or butt roast
- 1 cup BBQ sauce
- 1/2 cup chicken broth
- 2 tablespoons brown sugar
- 1 tablespoon Worcestershire sauce
- 1 teaspoon smoked paprika
- Salt and pepper to taste
- Sandwich buns
- Coleslaw for topping (optional)

*Instructions:*

- ✓ Season pork shoulder or butt roast with salt, pepper, and smoked paprika.
- ✓ In a bowl, put together the BBQ sauce, chicken broth, brown sugar, and Worcestershire sauce.
- ✓ Place the seasoned pork in a slow cooker and pour the BBQ sauce mixture over it.
- ✓ Cover and cook on low for 6-8 hours or until pork is tender and easily shreds with a fork.

✓ Remove the pork from the slow cooker and shred it using two forks.

✓ Make sure to return the shredded pork to the slow cooker and mix it with the sauce.

✓ Serve the BBQ pulled pork on sandwich buns, topped with coleslaw if desired.

*Nutritional Information:*

*Calories: 380 | Protein: 25g | Fat: 15g | Carbs: 30g | Fiber: 2g*

## Beef and Vegetable Stir-Fry

**Servings: 4 | Prep Time: 15 mins | Cooking Time: 15 mins**

*Ingredients:*

- 1 lb. beef sirloin, thinly and finely sliced
- 2 tablespoons soy sauce
- 2 tablespoons oyster sauce
- 2 tablespoons hoisin sauce
- 1 tablespoon sesame oil
- 2 cloves garlic, minced
- 1 teaspoon grated ginger
- 2 cups mixed vegetables, sliced
- Cooked rice or noodles for serving

- Sesame seeds and chopped green onions (used for garnishing)

*Instructions:*

- ✓ In a bowl, put together the soy sauce, oyster sauce, hoisin sauce, sesame oil, minced garlic, and grated ginger.
- ✓ Marinate thinly sliced beef in the sauce mixture for 10-15 minutes.
- ✓ Heat a wok or skillet over high heat. Add a bit of oil.
- ✓ Stir-fry marinated beef for 2-3 minutes until browned. Gently remove from the skillet and put it aside.
- ✓ In the same skillet, stir-fry mixed vegetables until tender-crisp.
- ✓ Return the cooked beef to the skillet and toss with the vegetables.
- ✓ Cook for an additional minute until everything is heated through and coated in the sauce.
- ✓ Serve this delightful beef and vegetable stir-fry over cooked rice or noodles.
- ✓ Garnish with sesame seeds and chopped green onions.

*Nutritional Information:*

*Calories: 320 | Protein: 30g | Fat: 12g | Carbs: 25g | Fiber: 4g*

# Balsamic Glazed Chicken Thighs

**Servings: 4 | Prep Time: 10 mins | Cooking Time: 25 mins**

*Ingredients:*

- 4 bone-in, skin-on chicken thighs
- Salt and pepper to taste
- 1/4 cup balsamic vinegar
- 2 tablespoons honey
- 2 cloves garlic, minced
- 1 tablespoon olive oil
- Chopped fresh parsley for garnish

*Instructions:*

- ✓ Set the temperature of the oven to 400°F (200°C).
- ✓ Adjust the chicken thighs with a little salt and pepper.
- ✓ Heat olive oil in an oven-proof skillet over moderate to high heat.
- ✓ Add chicken thighs to the skillet, skin-side down, and cook for 5-6 minutes until browned.
- ✓ Flip the chicken thighs and transfer the skillet to the preheated oven.
- ✓ Roast for 15-20 minutes or until the chicken is cooked through.

✓ Meanwhile, in a small saucepan, combine balsamic vinegar, honey, and minced garlic. Gently bring to a simmer and cook until everything is slightly thickened.

✓ Brush the balsamic glaze over the cooked chicken thighs.

✓ Nicely garnish with chopped fresh parsley before serving.

*Nutritional Information:*

*Calories: 280 | Protein: 25g | Fat: 18g | Carbs: 8g | Fiber: 0g*

# Turkey Chili

**Servings: 6 | Prep Time: 15 mins | Cooking Time: 30 mins**

*Ingredients:*

- 1 lb. ground turkey
- 1 onion, chopped
- 2 cloves garlic, minced
- 1 bell pepper, chopped
- 1 can (15 oz) diced tomatoes
- 1 can (15 oz) kidney beans, washed and drained
- 2 cups chicken broth
- 2 tablespoons chili powder
- 1 teaspoon cumin
- Salt and pepper to taste

- Shredded cheese and chopped cilantro (used for garnishing)

*Instructions:*

✓ In a large pot or Dutch oven, cook ground turkey until browned.

✓ Add chopped onion, minced garlic, and chopped bell pepper. Sauté until vegetables are tender.

✓ Stir in diced tomatoes, kidney beans, chicken broth, chili powder, cumin, salt, and pepper.

✓ Bring the mixture to a boil, then reduce heat and let it simmer for 20-25 minutes.

✓ Adjust seasoning if needed.

✓ Serve this hearty turkey chili topped with shredded cheese and chopped cilantro.

*Nutritional Information:*

*Calories: 280 | Protein: 20g | Fat: 8g | Carbs: 30g | Fiber: 8g*

# Italian Sausage Pasta

**Servings: 4 | Prep Time: 10 mins | Cooking Time: 20 mins**

*Ingredients:*

- 8 oz pasta of your choice
- 4 Italian sausage links, casings removed

- 1 onion, diced
- 2 cloves garlic, minced
- 1 can (14 oz) diced tomatoes
- 1/2 cup chicken broth
- 1 teaspoon dried basil
- 1 teaspoon dried oregano
- Salt and pepper to taste
- Grated Parmesan cheese for garnish
- Chopped fresh basil for garnish

*Instructions:*

✓ Cook pasta in accordance with the package instructions. Drain and set aside.

✓ In a skillet, cook Italian sausage over medium heat, breaking it into crumbles, until browned. Gently remove from the skillet and put it aside.

✓ In the same skillet, sauté diced onion until translucent. Continue to add minced garlic and cook until fragrant.

✓ Stir in diced tomatoes, chicken broth, dried basil, dried oregano, salt, and pepper. Simmer for 5 minutes.

✓ Return the cooked Italian sausage to the skillet and simmer for an additional 5 minutes.

✓ Toss cooked pasta with the sausage and tomato sauce.

✓ Serve this flavorful Italian sausage pasta, garnished with grated Parmesan cheese and chopped fresh basil.

*Nutritional Information:*

*Calories: 420 | Protein: 18g | Fat: 15g | Carbs: 50g | Fiber: 4g*

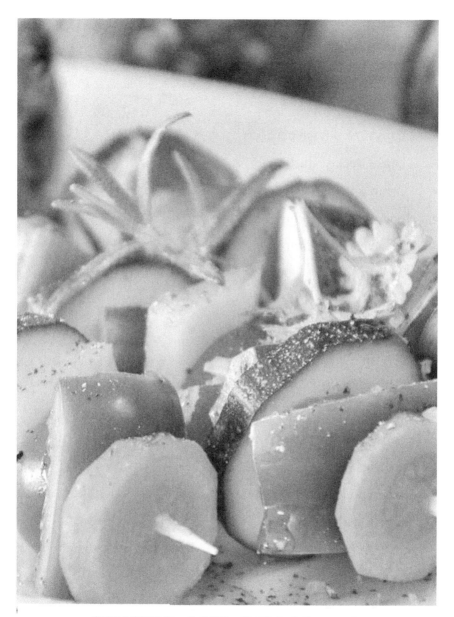

# FRUITS AND DESSERTS

# Fresh Berry Parfait

**Servings: 4 | Prep Time: 10 mins | Assembly Time: 5 mins**

*Ingredients:*

- 2 cups mixed fresh berries
- 2 cups Greek yogurt
- 1/2 cup granola
- Honey or maple syrup (optional)
- Mint leaves for garnish

*Instructions:*

- ✓ Wash and prepare the fresh berries by slicing strawberries if needed.
- ✓ In serving glasses or bowls, layer Greek yogurt, fresh berries, and granola.
- ✓ Repeat the layers until the glasses are filled, ending with a layer of berries on top.
- ✓ Drizzle honey or maple syrup for extra sweetness if desired.
- ✓ Garnish with mint leaves.
- ✓ Serve these delightful fresh berry parfaits immediately as a healthy and satisfying dessert or breakfast option.

*Nutritional Information:*

*Calories: 220 | Protein: 10g | Fat: 5g | Carbs: 35g | Fiber: 5g*

# Grilled Pineapple with Cinnamon

**Servings: 4 | Prep Time: 5 mins | Grilling Time: 8 mins**

*Ingredients:*

- 1 pineapple, peeled and carefully sliced into rings
- 2 tablespoons honey
- 1 teaspoon ground cinnamon

*Instructions:*

- ✓ Preheat the grill or grill pan over moderate to high heat.
- ✓ Brush pineapple rings with honey on both sides.
- ✓ Place pineapple rings on the grill and cook for about 4 minutes on each side until grill marks appear.
- ✓ Remove from the grill and sprinkle ground cinnamon over the grilled pineapple rings.
- ✓ Serve these caramelized grilled pineapple slices as a delightful dessert or alongside a main dish.

*Nutritional Information:*

*Calories: 90 | Protein: 1g | Fat: 0g | Carbs: 25g | Fiber: 3g*

# Mango Coconut Chia Pudding

**Servings: 4 | Prep Time: 5 mins | Chilling Time: 4 hrs.**

*Ingredients:*

- 1 cup diced ripe mango
- 1 can (13.5 oz) coconut milk
- 1/4 cup chia seeds
- 2 tablespoons honey or agave syrup
- 1 teaspoon vanilla extract

*Instructions:*

- ✓ In a blender, puree diced mango until smooth.
- ✓ In a mixing bowl, put together the coconut milk, chia seeds, honey or agave syrup, and vanilla extract.
- ✓ Stir in the mango puree and mix well.
- ✓ Cover and refrigerate for at least 4 hours or overnight until the chia pudding thickens.
- ✓ Serve this creamy and tropical mango coconut chia pudding chilled, optionally topped with additional diced mango.

*Nutritional Information:*

*Calories: 250 | Protein: 4g | Fat: 20g | Carbs: 15g | Fiber: 6g*

# Baked Apples with Cinnamon

**Servings: 4 | Prep Time: 10 mins | Baking Time: 30 mins**

*Ingredients:*

- 4 apples, cored
- 2 tablespoons melted butter or coconut oil of your choice
- 2 tablespoons brown sugar (maple syrup is also preferable)
- 1 teaspoon ground cinnamon
- Chopped nuts or granola (used for topping)
- Greek yogurt or ice cream (used for serving)

*Instructions:*

- ✓ Set the temperature of the oven to 375°F (190°C).
- ✓ Place cored apples in a baking dish.
- ✓ In a bowl, put together the melted butter or coconut oil, brown sugar or maple syrup, and ground cinnamon.
- ✓ Spoon the mixture into the cores of the apples, distributing evenly.
- ✓ Bake for 25-30 minutes or until the apples are tender.
- ✓ Serve these aromatic baked apples warm, optionally topped with chopped nuts or granola and a dollop of Greek yogurt or ice cream.

*Nutritional Information:*

*Calories: 180 | Protein: 1g | Fat: 7g | Carbs: 30g | Fiber: 5g*

# Lemon Blueberry Bars

**Servings: 12 | Prep Time: 15 mins | Baking Time: 35 mins**

*Ingredients:*

- 1 cup all-purpose flour
- 1/2 cup rolled oats
- 1/2 cup brown sugar
- 1/4 teaspoon salt
- 1/2 cup unsalted butter, melted
- 1 cup blueberries
- Zest and juice of 1 lemon
- 2 tablespoons granulated sugar
- 2 tablespoons cornstarch

*Instructions:*

- ✓ Set the temperature of the oven to 350°F (175°C). Make sure to line an 8x8-inch baking pan with parchment paper.
- ✓ In a mixing bowl, put together the flour, rolled oats, brown sugar, salt, and melted butter. Mix until crumbly.
- ✓ Press two-thirds of the mixture evenly into the bottom of the prepared baking pan to form the crust.
- ✓ In another bowl, toss blueberries with lemon zest, lemon juice, granulated sugar, and cornstarch.
- ✓ Spread the blueberry mixture over the crust in the baking pan.

✓ Sprinkle the remaining oat mixture evenly over the blueberry layer.

✓ Bake for 35 minutes or until the top is golden brown.

✓ Allow the lemon blueberry bars to cool completely before slicing into squares.

*Nutritional Information:*

*Calories: 160 | Protein: 2g | Fat: 7g | Carbs: 23g | Fiber: 1g*

# Mixed Fruit Salad

**Servings: 6 | Prep Time: 15 mins | Cooking Time: 0 min**

*Ingredients:*

- 2 cups cubed watermelon
- 2 cups cubed cantaloupe
- 2 cups cubed honeydew melon
- 1 cup halved grapes
- 1 cup sliced strawberries
- 1/4 cup fresh mint leaves, chopped
- Juice of 1 lime
- 2 tablespoons honey or maple syrup
- Optional: shredded coconut for garnish

*Instructions:*

✓ In a large mixing bowl, put together the watermelon, cantaloupe, honeydew melon, grapes, strawberries, and chopped mint leaves.

✓ In a small bowl, whisk together lime juice and honey or maple syrup to make the dressing.

✓ Drizzle the dressing over the fruit salad and toss gently to coat.

✓ Chill the mixed fruit salad in the refrigerator for at least 30 minutes before serving.

✓ Serve this refreshing mixed fruit salad garnished with shredded coconut if desired.

*Nutritional Information:*

*Calories: 90 | Protein: 1g | Fat: 0g | Carbs: 23g | Fiber: 2g*

# Chocolate-Dipped Strawberries

**Servings: 6 | Prep Time: 15 mins | Cooking Time: 30 mins**

*Ingredients:*

- 12 large strawberries, washed and dried
- 4 oz dark or milk chocolate, nicely chopped
- 1 teaspoon coconut oil or vegetable shortening (optional)

*Instructions:*

✓ Line a baking sheet with parchment paper.

✓ In a microwave-safe bowl, melt the chopped chocolate in 30-second intervals, stirring until smooth. Add coconut oil or vegetable shortening if desired for a smoother consistency.

✓ Hold each strawberry by the stem and dip it into the melted chocolate, covering about two-thirds of the strawberry.

✓ Place the chocolate-dipped strawberries on the prepared baking sheet.

✓ Chill the strawberries in the refrigerator for at least 30 minutes or until the chocolate is set.

✓ Serve these delightful chocolate-dipped strawberries as a sweet treat or dessert.

*Nutritional Information:*

*Calories: 70 | Protein: 1g | Fat: 4g | Carbs: 10g | Fiber: 2g*

# Pineapple Upside-Down Cake

**Servings: 8 | Prep Time: 20 mins | Baking Time: 45 mins**

*Ingredients:*

● 1/4 cup unsalted butter

● 1/2 cup brown sugar

- 8 pineapple rings (canned or fresh)
- 8 maraschino cherries
- 1 1/2 cups all-purpose flour
- 1 cup granulated sugar
- 1 teaspoon baking powder
- 1/2 teaspoon baking soda
- 1/2 teaspoon salt
- 1/2 cup unsweetened applesauce
- 1/2 cup buttermilk
- 1/4 cup vegetable oil
- 1 teaspoon vanilla extract

*Instructions:*

✓ Set the temperature of the oven to 350°F (175°C). Grease a round 9-inch cake pan.

✓ Melt butter and brown sugar together. Gently spread the mixture evenly in the cake pan.

✓ Arrange pineapple rings over the butter-sugar mixture and place a cherry in the center of each ring.

✓ In a mixing bowl, put together the flour, granulated sugar, baking powder, baking soda, and salt.

✓ Add applesauce, buttermilk, vegetable oil, and vanilla extract to the dry ingredients. Mix until just combined.

✓ Pour the batter over the pineapple in the cake pan.

✓ Bake for 40-45 minutes or until a toothpick inserted into the center comes out clean.

✓ Allow the pineapple upside-down cake to cool in the pan for 10 minutes before inverting it onto a serving plate.

*Nutritional Information:*

*Calories: 320 | Protein: 3g | Fat: 10g | Carbs: 55g | Fiber: 1g*

# Banana Bread

**Servings: 10 | Prep Time: 15 mins | Baking Time: 60 mins**

*Ingredients:*

- 2 cups all-purpose flour
- 1 teaspoon baking soda
- 1/4 teaspoon salt
- 1/2 cup unsalted butter, softened
- 3/4 cup brown sugar
- 2 large eggs
- 4 ripe bananas, mashed
- 1/3 cup plain Greek yogurt (sour cream also preferable)
- 1 teaspoon vanilla extract
- Optional: chopped nuts or chocolate chips

*Instructions:*

✓ Set the temperature of the oven to 350°F (175°C). Grease a 9x5-inch loaf pan.

✓ In a mixing bowl, whisk together flour, baking soda, and salt.

✓ In a separate bowl, cream together softened butter and brown sugar until light and fluffy.

✓ Beat in eggs, mashed bananas, Greek yogurt or sour cream, and vanilla extract until well combined.

✓ Now, you can gradually add the dry ingredients to the wet ingredients, mixing until just combined. Do not overmix.

✓ If desired, fold in chopped nuts or chocolate chips into the batter.

✓ Gently transfer the batter into the prepared loaf pan and smooth the top.

✓ Bake for 50-60 minutes or until a toothpick inserted into the center comes out clean.

✓ Allow the banana bread to cool in the pan for 10-15 minutes before transferring it to a wire rack to cool completely.

*Nutritional Information:*

*Calories: 280 | Protein: 4g | Fat: 11g | Carbs: 42g | Fiber: 2g*

## Raspberry Lemon Loaf

**Servings: 8 | Prep Time: 15 mins | Baking Time: 50 mins**

*Ingredients:*

- 1 1/2 cups all-purpose flour
- 1 1/2 teaspoons baking powder
- 1/4 teaspoon salt
- 1/2 cup unsalted butter, softened
- 3/4 cup granulated sugar
- 2 large eggs
- Zest and juice of 1 lemon
- 1/2 cup plain Greek yogurt
- 1 cup fresh raspberries
- Optional: powdered sugar for dusting

*Instructions:*

- ✓ Set the temperature of the oven to 350°F (175°C). Grease a 9x5-inch loaf pan.
- ✓ In a bowl, gently whisk together the flour, the baking powder, and the salt.
- ✓ In another bowl, cream together softened butter and granulated sugar until light and fluffy.
- ✓ Beat in eggs, lemon zest, and lemon juice until well combined.
- ✓ Gradually add the dry ingredients to the wet ingredients, alternating with Greek yogurt, mixing until just combined.
- ✓ Gently fold in fresh raspberries.

✓ Gently transfer the batter into the prepared loaf pan and smooth the top.

✓ Bake for 45-50 minutes or until a toothpick inserted into the center comes out clean.

✓ Let the raspberry lemon loaf cool in the pan for 10 minutes before transferring it to a wire rack to cool completely.

✓ Dust with powdered sugar before serving if you prefer.

*Nutritional Information:*

*Calories: 280 | Protein: 5g | Fat: 12g | Carbs: 38g | Fiber: 2g*

## Apple Crisp

**Servings: 6 | Prep Time: 15 mins | Baking Time: 45 mins**

*Ingredients:*

- 4 cups sliced apples (peeled and cored)
- 1 tablespoon lemon juice
- 1/4 cup granulated sugar
- 1 teaspoon ground cinnamon
- 1/2 cup old-fashioned rolled oats
- 1/2 cup all-purpose flour
- 1/4 cup brown sugar
- 1/4 cup unsalted butter, cold and cubed

- Vanilla ice cream or whipped cream for serving (optional)

*Instructions:*

✓ Set the temperature of the oven to 350°F (175°C). Grease a baking dish.

✓ In a bowl, toss sliced apples with lemon juice, granulated sugar, and ground cinnamon. Make sure to spread evenly in the prepared baking dish.

✓ In another bowl, put together the rolled oats, flour, brown sugar, and cubed cold butter. Use your fingers or a fork to create a crumbly mixture.

✓ Sprinkle the oat mixture evenly over the apples in the baking dish.

✓ Bake for forty (40) to forty-five (45) minutes or until the topping is golden brown and the apples are tender.

✓ Serve this comforting apple crisp warm, optionally topped with vanilla ice cream or whipped cream.

*Nutritional Information:*

*Calories: 220 | Protein: 2g | Fat: 9g | Carbs: 36g | Fiber: 4g*

# Chocolate Avocado Mousse

**Servings: 4 | Prep Time: 10 mins | Chilling Time: 60 mins**

*Ingredients:*

- 2 ripe avocados, peeled and pitted
- 1/4 cup cocoa powder
- 1/4 cup honey or maple syrup
- 1 teaspoon vanilla extract
- Pinch of salt
- Optional: fresh berries for garnish

*Instructions:*

- ✓ In a blender or food processor, blend avocados, cocoa powder, honey or maple syrup, vanilla extract, and a pinch of salt until smooth and creamy.
- ✓ Divide the chocolate avocado mousse into serving dishes.
- ✓ Make sure to chill in the refrigerator for at least one hour before serving.
- ✓ Garnish with fresh berries before serving if desired.

*Nutritional Information:*

*Calories: 200 | Protein: 3g | Fat: 13g | Carbs: 24g | Fiber: 7g*

# Blueberry Lemon Scones

**Servings: 8 | Prep Time: 15 mins | Baking Time: 20 mins**

*Ingredients:*

- 2 cups all-purpose flour
- 1/4 cup granulated sugar
- 1 tablespoon baking powder
- Zest of 1 lemon
- 1/2 teaspoon salt
- 1/2 cup unsalted butter, cold and cubed
- 1 cup fresh blueberries
- 2/3 cup heavy cream
- 1 teaspoon vanilla extract
- Optional: coarse sugar for sprinkling

*Instructions:*

- ✓ Set the temperature of the oven to 400°F (200°C). Make sure to line a baking sheet with parchment paper.
- ✓ In a bowl, whisk together flour, granulated sugar, baking powder, lemon zest, and salt.
- ✓ Add cold, cubed butter to the flour mixture and use a pastry cutter or two knives to cut the butter into the dry ingredients until it resembles coarse crumbs.
- ✓ Gently fold in fresh blueberries.

✓ In a separate bowl, put together the heavy cream and vanilla extract.

✓ Gradually add the cream mixture to the dry ingredients, stirring until just combined.

✓ Turn the dough out onto a floured surface and pat it into a circle about 1-inch thick.

✓ Cut the dough into 8 wedges and place them on the prepared baking sheet.

✓ Optional: Sprinkle the tops of the scones with coarse sugar for added sweetness and texture.

✓ Now, bake for eighteen (18) to twenty (20) minutes or until golden brown.

✓ Allow the blueberry lemon scones to cool on a wire rack before serving.

*Nutritional Information:*

*Calories: 290 | Protein: 4g | Fat: 15g | Carbs: 36g | Fiber: 1g*

# Peach Cobbler

**Servings: 6 | Prep Time: 15 mins | Baking Time: 45 mins**

*Ingredients:*

- 4 cups sliced fresh or canned peaches
- 1/2 cup granulated sugar

- 1 tablespoon lemon juice
- 1 teaspoon vanilla extract
- 1/2 teaspoon ground cinnamon
- 1 cup all-purpose flour
- 1/2 cup granulated sugar
- 1 teaspoon baking powder
- 1/4 teaspoon salt
- 1/2 cup unsalted butter, melted
- Vanilla ice cream for serving (optional)

*Instructions:*

✓ Set the temperature of the oven to 375°F (190°C). Grease a baking dish.

✓ In a bowl, put together the sliced peaches, granulated sugar, lemon juice, vanilla extract, and ground cinnamon. Toss to coat the peaches evenly.

✓ Spread the peach mixture in the prepared baking dish.

✓ In another bowl, mix the flour, granulated sugar, baking powder, and salt.

✓ Stir in melted butter until a crumbly mixture form.

✓ Evenly distribute the flour-butter mixture over the peaches in the baking dish.

✓ Bake for 40-45 minutes or until the topping is golden brown and the filling is bubbly.

✓ Serve this classic peach cobbler warm, optionally topped with vanilla ice cream.

*Nutritional Information:*

*Calories: 330 | Protein: 2g | Fat: 14g | Carbs: 51g | Fiber: 3g*

## Lemon Ricotta Pancakes

**Servings: 4 | Prep Time: 10 mins | Cooking Time: 15 mins**

*Ingredients:*

- 1 cup all-purpose flour
- 2 tablespoons granulated sugar
- 1 teaspoon baking powder
- 1/2 teaspoon baking soda
- 1/4 teaspoon salt
- 1 cup ricotta cheese
- 2 large eggs
- 3/4 cup milk
- Zest and juice of 1 lemon
- Butter or oil for cooking
- Maple syrup and fresh berries for serving

*Instructions:*

- ✓ In a bowl, whisk together flour, sugar, baking powder, baking soda, and salt.
- ✓ In another bowl, combine the ricotta cheese, eggs, milk, lemon zest, and lemon juice. Mix until smooth.
- ✓ Gradually add the wet ingredients to the dry ingredients, stirring until just combined. Make sure you do not overmix; some lumps are okay.
- ✓ Heat a griddle or skillet over moderate heat and lightly grease with butter or oil.
- ✓ Pour 1/4 cup portions of batter onto the griddle and cook until bubbles form on the surface. Flip and cook until golden brown.
- ✓ Repeat with the remaining batter.
- ✓ Serve these fluffy lemon ricotta pancakes warm, topped with maple syrup and fresh berries.

*Nutritional Information:*

*Calories: 290 | Protein: 11g | Fat: 10g | Carbs: 38g | Fiber: 1g*

# Strawberry Shortcake

**Servings: 6 | Prep Time: 20 mins | Baking Time: 15 mins**

*Ingredients:*

- 2 cups sliced strawberries
- 2 tablespoons granulated sugar
- 2 cups all-purpose flour
- 1/4 cup granulated sugar
- 1 tablespoon baking powder
- 1/2 teaspoon salt
- 1/2 cup unsalted butter, cold and cubed
- 3/4 cup milk
- Whipped cream for serving

*Instructions:*

- ✓ In a bowl, toss sliced strawberries with granulated sugar. Set aside to macerate.
- ✓ Set the temperature of the oven to 425°F (220°C). Make sure to line a baking sheet with parchment paper.
- ✓ In a mixing bowl, whisk together the flour, sugar, baking powder, and salt.
- ✓ Cut in cold, cubed butter using a pastry cutter or two knives until the mixture resembles coarse crumbs.
- ✓ Gradually add milk, mixing until the dough comes together.

✓ Turn the dough out onto a floured surface and pat it into a circle about 3/4-inch thick.

✓ Use a biscuit cutter or glass to cut out circles of dough and place them on the prepared baking sheet.

✓ Now, bake for twelve (12) to fifteen (15) minutes or until golden brown.

✓ Split the baked shortcakes in half horizontally.

✓ Spoon macerated strawberries onto the bottom halves, top with whipped cream, and cover with the top halves of the shortcakes.

✓ Serve these delightful strawberry shortcakes immediately.

*Nutritional Information:*

*Calories: 320 | Protein: 5g | Fat: 14g | Carbs: 44g | Fiber: 2g*

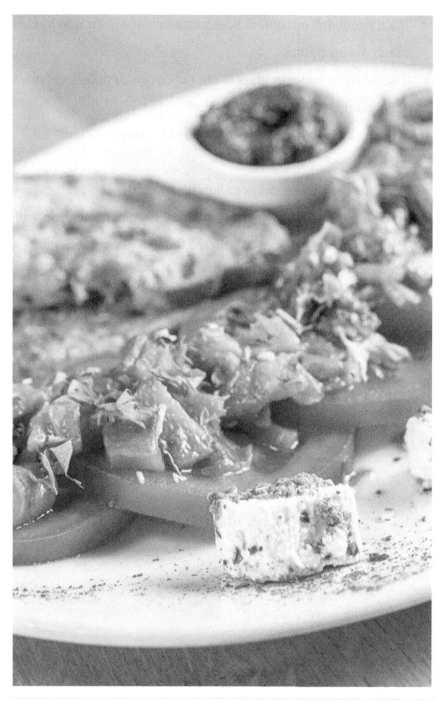

# 30-DAY

# MEAL

# PLAN

## KEY

**A- BREAKFAST**

**B- LUNCH**

**C- DINNER**

| DAY | A | B | C |
|---|---|---|---|
| 1 | Avocado Toast with Poached Egg | Quinoa Salad with Chickpeas and Veggies | Grilled Salmon with Lemon-Dill Sauce, Roasted Sweet Potatoes, Steamed Broccoli |
| 2 | Greek Yogurt Parfait with Fresh Berries | Turkey and Avocado Wrap with a Side of Mixed Greens | Spaghetti with Tomato Basil Sauce, Turkey Meatballs, and Whole Wheat Pasta |
| 3 | Blueberry Chia Seed Pudding | Mediterranean Chickpea Salad | Chicken Stir-Fry with Brown Rice and Mixed Vegetables |
| 4 | Mixed Fruit Smoothie with Spinach and Greek Yogurt | Lentil and Vegetable Soup | Baked Cod with Quinoa Pilaf, Roasted Brussels Sprouts |
| 5 | Oatmeal with Sliced Banana and Almonds | Caprese Salad with Whole Grain Baguette | Beef and Vegetable Skewers with Couscous, Grilled Zucchini |

| DAY | | | |
|---|---|---|---|
| 6 | Whole Wheat Pancakes with Fresh Berries | Hummus and Veggie Wrap | Shrimp and Vegetable Stir-Fry with Brown Rice |
| 7 | Yogurt and Berry Smoothie Bowl | Quinoa and Black Bean Bowl with Avocado | Grilled Chicken Breast with Quinoa Salad, Steamed Asparagus |
| 8 | Banana Walnut Muffins | Tuna Salad Lettuce Wraps | Vegetarian Chili with Whole Grain Bread |
| 9 | Strawberry Banana Overnight Oats | Turkey and Vegetable Stir-Fry with Brown Rice | Baked Eggplant Parmesan with Whole Wheat Spaghetti |
| 10 | Spinach and Feta Omelet | Chickpea and Spinach Stuffed Sweet Potatoes | Grilled Swordfish with Quinoa and Roasted Vegetables |

| DAY | | | |
|---|---|---|---|
| 11 | Lemon Blueberry Bars | Mixed Fruit Salad with Lime-Honey Dressing | Chocolate-Dipped Strawberries as a sweet treat after Grilled Chicken Salad |
| 12 | Mango Coconut Chia Pudding | Greek Salad with Grilled Shrimp | Pineapple Upside-Down Cake for dessert after Vegetable Stir-Fry with Tofu |
| 13 | Baked Apples with Cinnamon | Lemon Ricotta Pancakes with Maple Syrup and Berries | Strawberry Shortcake for dessert after Baked Cod with Quinoa Pilaf |
| 14 | Blueberry Lemon Scones | Chicken Caesar Salad Wrap | Lemon Garlic Roast Chicken with Roasted Vegetables |
| 15 | Peach Cobbler Smoothie | Caprese Sandwich with a Side of Mixed Greens | Turkey and Vegetable Skewers with Couscous, Grilled Zucchini |

| DAY | A | B | C |
|---|---|---|---|
| 16 | Chocolate Avocado Mousse | Quinoa and Black Bean Bowl with Avocado | Beef and Vegetable Stir-Fry with Brown Rice |
| 17 | Strawberry Banana Smoothie with Spinach | Mediterranean Chickpea Salad | Shrimp Scampi with Whole Wheat Pasta and Steamed Broccoli |
| 18 | Banana Bread Slices | Hummus and Veggie Wrap | Eggplant and Chickpea Curry with Brown Rice |
| 19 | Raspberry Lemon Loaf | Tuna Salad Lettuce Wraps | Grilled Swordfish with Quinoa and Roasted Vegetables |
| 20 | Lemon Ricotta Pancakes | Lentil and Vegetable Soup | Baked Eggplant Parmesan with Whole Wheat Spaghetti |

| DAY | A | B | C |
|-----|---|---|---|
| 21 | Mixed Fruit Smoothie with Spinach and Greek Yogurt | Quinoa Salad with Chickpeas and Veggies | Grilled Salmon with Lemon-Dill Sauce, Roasted Sweet Potatoes, Steamed Broccoli |
| 22 | Blueberry Chia Seed Pudding | Turkey and Avocado Wrap with a Side of Mixed Greens | Baked Cod with Quinoa Pilaf, Roasted Brussels Sprouts |
| 23 | Avocado Toast with Poached Egg | Quinoa and Black Bean Bowl with Avocado | Chocolate-Dipped Strawberries after Chicken Stir-Fry with Brown Rice |
| 24 | Strawberry Banana Overnight Oats | Caprese Salad with Whole Grain Baguette | Grilled Swordfish with Quinoa and Roasted Vegetables |
| 25 | Lemon Blueberry Bars | Greek Salad with Grilled Shrimp | Beef and Vegetable Stir-Fry with Brown Rice |

| DAY | A | B | C |
|---|---|---|---|
| 26 | Oatmeal with Sliced Banana and Almonds | Lentil and Vegetable Soup | Baked Eggplant Parmesan with Whole Wheat Spaghetti |
| 27 | Yogurt and Berry Smoothie Bowl | Mediterranean Chickpea Salad | Shrimp Scampi with Whole Wheat Pasta and Steamed Broccoli |
| 28 | Banana Bread Slices | Tuna Salad Lettuce Wraps | Grilled Salmon with Lemon-Dill Sauce, Roasted Sweet Potatoes, Steamed Broccoli |
| 29 | Chocolate Avocado Mousse | Hummus and Veggie Wrap | Vegetable Stir-Fry with Tofu, followed by Strawberry Shortcake |
| 30 | Lemon Ricotta Pancakes | Chickpea and Spinach Stuffed Sweet Potatoes | Baked Chicken Breast with Quinoa Salad, Steamed Asparagus |

# Weekly Meal Planner

| WEEKS | BREAKFAST | LUNCH | DINNER |
|-------|-----------|-------|--------|
| MON | | | |
| TUE | | | |
| WED | | | |
| THU | | | |
| FRI | | | |
| SAT | | | |
| SUN | | | |

# Weekly Meal Planner

| WEEKS | BREAKFAST | LUNCH | DINNER |
|-------|-----------|-------|--------|
| MON | | | |
| TUE | | | |
| WED | | | |
| THU | | | |
| FRI | | | |
| SAT | | | |
| SUN | | | |

# Weekly Meal Planner

| WEEKS | BREAKFAST | LUNCH | DINNER |
|-------|-----------|-------|--------|
| MON | | | |
| TUE | | | |
| WED | | | |
| THU | | | |
| FRI | | | |
| SAT | | | |
| SUN | | | |

# Weekly Meal Planner

| WEEKS | BREAKFAST | LUNCH | DINNER |
|-------|-----------|-------|--------|
| MON | | | |
| TUE | | | |
| WED | | | |
| THU | | | |
| FRI | | | |
| SAT | | | |
| SUN | | | |

# Weekly Meal Planner

| WEEKS | BREAKFAST | LUNCH | DINNER |
|-------|-----------|-------|--------|
| MON | | | |
| TUE | | | |
| WED | | | |
| THU | | | |
| FRI | | | |
| SAT | | | |
| SUN | | | |

# Weekly Meal Planner

| WEEKS | BREAKFAST | LUNCH | DINNER |
|-------|-----------|-------|--------|
| MON   |           |       |        |
| TUE   |           |       |        |
| WED   |           |       |        |
| THU   |           |       |        |
| FRI   |           |       |        |
| SAT   |           |       |        |
| SUN   |           |       |        |

## Weekly Meal Planner

| WEEKS | BREAKFAST | LUNCH | DINNER |
|-------|-----------|-------|--------|
| MON | | | |
| TUE | | | |
| WED | | | |
| THU | | | |
| FRI | | | |
| SAT | | | |
| SUN | | | |

## NOTES

## NOTES

## NOTES

_____

_____

_____

_____

_____

_____

_____

_____

_____

_____

_____

_____

_____

_____

_____

_____

_____

_____

_____

_____

_____

_____

_____

_____

_____

_____

## NOTES

_____
_____
_____
_____
_____
_____
_____
_____
_____
_____
_____
_____
_____
_____
_____
_____
_____
_____
_____
_____
_____
_____
_____
_____

## NOTES

## NOTES

_____
_____
_____
_____
_____
_____
_____
_____
_____
_____
_____
_____
_____
_____
_____
_____
_____
_____
_____
_____
_____
_____
_____

## NOTES

## NOTES

_____

_____

_____

_____

_____

_____

_____

_____

_____

_____

_____

_____

_____

_____

_____

_____

_____

_____

_____

_____

_____

_____

_____

_____

## NOTES

_____
_____
_____
_____
_____
_____
_____
_____
_____
_____
_____
_____
_____
_____
_____
_____
_____
_____
_____
_____
_____
_____
_____
_____
_____

## NOTES

_____

_____

_____

_____

_____

_____

_____

_____

_____

_____

_____

_____

_____

_____

_____

_____

_____

_____

_____

_____

_____

_____

_____

_____

_____

_____

_____

_____

# NOTES

_____

_____

_____

_____

_____

_____

_____

_____

_____

_____

_____

_____

_____

_____

_____

_____

_____

_____

_____

_____

_____

_____

_____

_____

_____

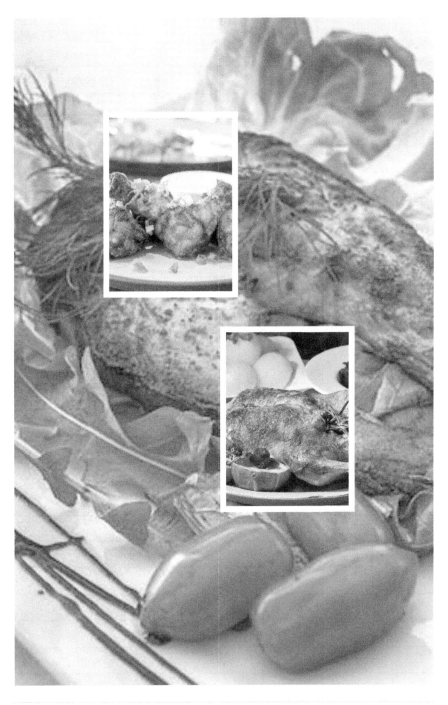

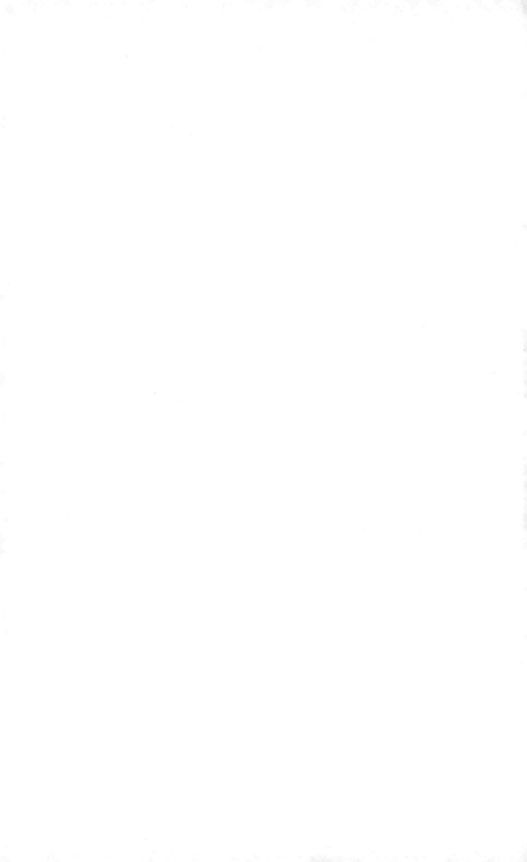

Made in the USA
Columbia, SC
11 April 2024

34232664R00108